I0473968

OVERCOMING BLADDER DISEASE

A Strategic Plan for Research

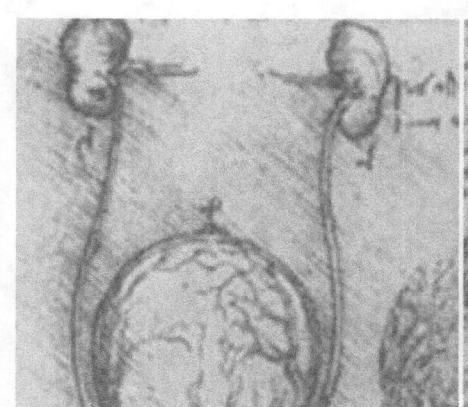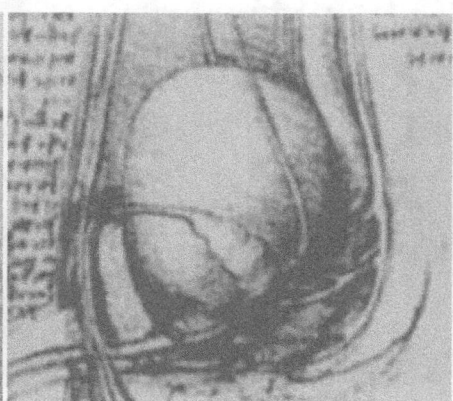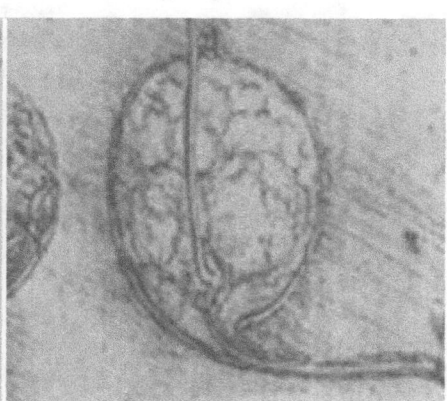

A REPORT OF THE BLADDER RESEARCH PROGRESS REVIEW GROUP

National Institute of Diabetes & Digestive & Kidney Diseases

National Institutes of Health

August 2002

TABLE OF CONTENTS

Letter from the Chair

I am pleased to present *Overcoming Bladder Disease: A Strategic Plan for Bladder Research*, developed by the Bladder Research Progress Review Group (BRPRG), to the Advisory Committee of the Director of the National Institute of Diabetes and Digestive and Kidney Diseases (NIDDK). The BRPRG's assessment of the Institute's progress in bladder research and strategic plan for future research was undertaken at the request of Dr. Allen Spiegel, director of the NIDDK. This strategic plan recommends future research directions and priorities and the means of implementing recommendations.

The BRPRG was an independent group of scientists and medical professionals who are prominent in clinical and basic research and professional and lay patient organizations related to the bladder. These colleagues represent the wide expertise required to assess the state of bladder research in the United States and to recommend research actions that could reduce morbidity and mortality of bladder diseases previously neglected. Such research has the potential for improving the quality of life of Americans with problems of the developing and aging urinary tract and with conditions such as urinary obstruction, interstitial cystitis, urinary tract infection, complications of diabetes, urinary incontinence, and cancer.

The BRPRG was composed of an Executive Committee and 14 subcommittees. In developing this plan, the Executive Committee had many discussions and held plenary meetings throughout 2001 with the objective of developing a strategic national plan for bladder research. The BRPRG analyzed and assessed ongoing scientific investigation relevant to the lower urinary tract, defined unmet needs in bladder research, and developed goals and recommendations for future research and its implementation.

This was a difficult task, and the hard work of the BRPRG is evident in this report. The report emphasizes the current deficiencies in research efforts related to bladder and the intense need for improvement in the resources designated for bladder research. Advances in biomedical science and technology have opened the door for rapid and significant advances in bladder research that will improve the diagnosis, management, and prevention of bladder problems for many Americans.

My colleagues and I thank the Institute and its leadership for their recognition of the need for assessing bladder research. We anticipate following the progress of the recommendations made in this report, and we will be pleased to discuss our findings with the leadership of the National Institute of Diabetes and Digestive and Kidney Diseases.

Respectfully submitted,

Linda M. Dairiki Shortliffe, M.D.

*Chair, Bladder Research
Progress Review Group*

Executive Committee

We, the undersigned members of the Bladder Research Progress Review Group
Executive Committee, concur with this report:

William de Groat. Ph.D.

Vicki Ratner. M.D.

John O. DeLancey, M.D.

Anthony J. Schaeffer. M.D.

Monica Liebert, Ph.D.

William D. Steers, M.D.

John D. McConnell, M.D.

Dana Weaver-Osterholtz, M.D.

ACKNOWLEDGEMENTS

Josephine P. Briggs, M.D., *Director, Division of Kidney, Urologic, and Hematologic Diseases (DKUH), National Institute of Diabetes and Digestive and Kidney Diseases (NIDDK),* was the Executive Director of the BRPRG. Her expertise, advice, and support contributed tremendously to the development of the Strategic Research Plan.

The BRPRG thanks numerous National Institutes of Health representatives who helped provide technical information and organizational support. In particular, **Leroy M. Nyberg**, **Ph.D.**, **M.D.**, *Director, Urology Program, NIDDK,* and **Monica Liebert**, **Ph.D.**, formerly, *Associate Director, Urology Research, NIDDK,* and currently, *Director of Research, American Urological Association.*

We thank **Mary Harris**, writer and editor, *Office of Communications, NIDDK,* for her outstanding organizing efforts and **Carolyn Benson**, writer and editor, *DKUH,* for her outstanding scientific writing and editing for this report.

The BRPRG also thanks the **American Urogynecologic Society**, **American Urological Association**, **National Bladder Foundation**, and the **National Institute on Aging** for co-sponsoring with the NIH the meeting at Xerox Park University.

EXECUTIVE SUMMARY AND RECOMMENDATIONS

Introduction

Diseases and conditions affecting the bladder and associated structures of the lower urinary tract are a leading cause of urinary incontinence, pelvic pain, and kidney failure, and they often contribute to poor quality of life. It has been estimated that 35 million Americans suffer from bladder disease and most have chronic conditions. Bladder problems have been reported to cost Americans more than $16 billion per year in health-related expenses, and this estimate does not take into account the associated physical and emotional disabilities that are considered "unmentionable" by many men, women, and children.

Benjamin Franklin documented the poor quality of life for people with bladder problems in 1752. He invented the first flexible urethral catheter, made of silver and covered with gut, to help his brother empty his bladder. Franklin's brother suffered from bladder outlet obstruction caused by bladder stones. Years later, Franklin, who suffered from the same problem, was forced to catheterize himself intermittently with his own invention.[1] (See page 199) Although technology now provides better instrumentation, medical science has not solved many cases of urinary retention—or other problems related to the bladder—and intermittent catheterization much as Franklin described is still used.

Bladder diseases and problems affect people of all ages, races, and ethnic groups. Even with access to the best medical care, many people still suffer bladder pain, urinary incontinence, and loss of bladder function that may damage the kidneys. Strides have been taken to improve diagnosis, management, and treatment of bladder diseases, but many primary questions about bladder formation, function, and disease remain. Moreover, although vital organs such as the heart, lungs, liver, kidneys, and pancreas have been successfully transplanted, medical science has been unable to transplant or totally replace the bladder.

The Bladder Research Progress Review Group (BRPRG) was formed by the National Institute of Diabetes and Digestive and Kidney Disease (NIDDK) of the National Institutes of Health (NIH) to examine the state of bladder research in the United States and to develop a plan for future research in this area. The members of the BRPRG are a multidisciplinary group of recognized experts in bladder research. Their task was a complex one because many diseases and conditions of the urinary tract such as incontinence, obstruction, interstitial cystitis, and spina bifida affect the bladder's structure and function. For instance, some conditions such as bladder exstrophy are primary and become lifelong health concerns. Other conditions such as bladder dysfunction resulting from diabetes, aging, or spinal cord injury are secondary and create acute and chronic medical problems. Still other conditions that primarily affect the nervous system or vascular systems, for example multiple sclerosis and Parkinson's disease, also affect the bladder. Bladder diseases such as bladder cancer or urinary tract infections affect specific tissues such as bladder epithelium; thus, research on these tissues will contribute directly to overall progress in cancer and infectious diseases research and not to research on bladder alone.

From early 2000 to July 2001, members of the BRPRG had discussions and intensive meetings to examine all areas of bladder-related problems categorized by diseases and by organ or tissue in an attempt to develop a strategic bladder research plan. This plan is provided in this document.

Overwhelmingly, the BRPRG has concluded that bladder research in the United States is inadequate, fraught with a number of impediments, and lags behind research in other areas that affect the health of Americans to a similar degree. The extent of health problems associated with the bladder emphasizes the urgent need to expand rapidly bladder health-related research not only to diagnose, manage, and treat bladder diseases, but also

[1] Kimbrough, HM. Benjamin Franklin (1706-1790). *Investig Urology.* 1975;12(6):509-10.

to discover the risk and preventive factors that will ultimately improve overall health. Recent discoveries and technological advances in biomedical science have provided a unique opportunity to make rapid and important advances in bladder research that might improve diagnosis, management, and prevention of bladder problems.

This report outlines future critical research on the basic science of the lower urinary tract and clinical studies of bladder diseases and conditions. It also makes specific recommendations for focused inclusion of biotechnologies that offer opportunities for bladder research. In addition, the report describes the kinds of programs that will provide a pipeline of new researchers through training, new collaborations, and infrastructure to support this work. The potential consequences of rapid progress in bladder research could save many children, women, and men from the physical and emotional consequences of bladder diseases and conditions.

The U.S. Investment in Bladder Health and Research

The U.S. Government, through the National Institutes of Health (NIH) will spend an estimated $67.8 million on bladder research in fiscal year 2002. This modest investment pales in comparison with the health and societal costs of bladder-associated problems to the U.S. economy. People with congenital and acquired bladder and urethral disease frequently have chronic problems that require long-term health care and that could lead to disease in other systems.

To allow bladder research to "catch up" with other research areas that have made dramatic advances over the past 20 years, a disproportionate investment must be made toward bladder research programs, training, and infrastructure.

NATIONAL INSTITUTES OF HEALTH URINARY BLADDER RESEARCH

(Dollars in Thousands)

Participating Institutes and Centers	FY 2002 Estimate
National Cancer Institute (NCI)	$31,300
National Heart, Lung, and Blood Institute (NHLBI)	195
National Institute of Diabetes and Digestive and Kidney Diseases (NIDDK)	14,300
National Institute of Neurological Disorders and Stroke (NINDS)	1,107
National Institute of Allergy and Infectious Diseases (NIAID)	4,737
National Institute of Child Health and Human Development (NICHD)	6,200
National Institute of Biomedical Imaging and Bioengineering (NIBIB)	1,235
National Institute of Environmental Health Sciences (NIEHS)	505
National Institute on Aging (NIA)	3,000
National Institute on Deafness and Other Communication Disorders (NIDCD)	60
National Center for Complementary and Alternative Medicine (NCCAM)	780
National Institute on Alcohol Abuse and Alcoholism (NIAAA)	2,371
National Center for Research Resources (NCRR)	1,194
National Institute of Nursing Research (NINR)	807
TOTAL (NIH)	**67,791**

Strategic Research Priorities

The bladder is a unique organ. The transitional epithelium that lines its inner surface and other parts of the lower urinary tract occurs nowhere else in the body. Although similar to other types of epithelial tissue, transitional epithelium has unique properties.

The bladder also has the unusual capability of allowing willful storage and emptying—a function that is quite different from other hollow organs such as the heart or stomach, neither of which is subject to this kind of voluntary control. As such, the bladder has unusual basic functions and properties that still need to be explored to allow better understanding of the mechanisms involved. The bladder, furthermore, offers a unique research environment; agents may be delivered into this hollow organ for measurement, absorption, adhesion, and potentially treatment.

The BRPRG has outlined the following specific areas in which strategic bladder research will make important contributions to basic scientific knowledge and to improved management and potential prevention of bladder diseases and conditions:

* New technology-driven basic and clinical research

* Focused research for basic systems and disease

* Epidemiology, outcomes evaluations, prevention, and bioethics

* Research infrastructure

Tremendous opportunity exists for rapid advances in bladder research if scientists explore and exploit new methodologies and technologies already used successfully in other areas. These tools, applied to basic research on the bladder, will allow new discoveries of the function of this unique organ and its tissues and will advance our understanding of bladder disease. Because these methodologies and technologies crosscut many areas of research, the BRPRG recommends that they be emphasized in strategies that foster bladder research development. Furthermore, the BRPRG recommends that future bladder research be based upon a stable and ongoing mechanism for recruiting, training, and retaining future investigators in this area.

New Technology-Driven Basic and Clinical Research

Clinical and basic bladder research could benefit from the rapidly emerging biotechnology discoveries in genomics, proteomics, and molecular and microarray technology. Rapidly developing pharmacologic discovery and computer technology open the door for clinical trials and database achievements that were not previously possible.

Focused Research for Basic Systems and Disease

Focused research plans should target improved management for persons with neurogenic bladder, developmental problems, diabetes, infection, inflammation, and obstruction. This report outlines research focused on (1) identifying and managing specific populations at risk for disease and its complications and (2) preventing these problems. Equally important is research to examine normal and abnormal bladder function and the contributions of nerves, blood vessels, muscles, connective tissues, and epithelium to general problems of the organ.

Epidemiology, Outcomes Evaluations, Prevention, and Bioethics

Clinical research is the cornerstone of health improvement for all Americans. Although basic research in the area of the bladder will increase our knowledge, this basic knowledge needs to be translated into active clinical research.

Research Infrastructure

Because past efforts in bladder research have been meager, the BRPRG recommends extraordinary support for rapidly increasing research projects, research programs, manpower training, and technology in the area of the bladder. In particular, investment in information technology is essential to make core resources such as biostatistics, bioinformatics, epidemiology, outcomes evaluations, and bioethics widely available

→ Develop new technology-driven basic and clinical research techniques, including

- Animal models (genetic knockout models)

- Stem cell therapy

- Gene therapy

- Tissue engineering

- Functional imaging

- Biomechanical and micro-engineering technology

- Genomics and proteomics

- Cell regulation

→ Develop focused research plans for basic systems and disease

→ Conduct studies that include epidemiology, outcomes evaluations, prevention, and bioethics

→ Establish a research infrastructure

Basic Science Advances and Opportunities

The BRPRG has outlined basic science areas in which bladder research can make important contributions to all areas of scientific research. Basic science areas include bladder epithelium, connective tissue, muscle, and nerves and blood vessels. These research priorities override disease boundaries. Although difficult to categorize, the BRPRG decided to group these research priorities according to tissue type even though it recognizes that many of these initiatives also crosscut tissue and organ areas.

→ Explore anatomic epithelial and transitional cell variation and function in the bladder

→ Examine regulation of normal and abnormal bladder epithelial cell growth and differentiation, specifically with relation to

- Gender

- Age

- Stretch

→ Identify epithelial-mesenchymal interactions

→ Determine cellular and molecular bases for epithelial disease and variation

→ Examine regulation of collagen deposition

→ Identify relationships of connective tissue to regeneration

→ Determine cell-matrix interactions with relation to cell-cell regulation, including

- Cell signaling

- Bladder development, function, mechanics, injury, and regeneration

→ Develop tissue, cell, and molecular imaging techniques

→ Determine characteristics of smooth and striated muscle physiology

→ Explore neuromodulation of bladder muscle

→ Examine receptor and effector pharmacology

→ Identify bladder muscle (detrusor) biomechanics

→ Explore brain imaging and bladder function

→ Improve basic knowledge of bladder neurophysiology —both mechanical motor and sensory function

→ Examine mechanisms involved in neural communication with the bladder

→ Explore mechanisms of nerve and vascular protection, preservation, and regeneration during aging, injury, and disease

→ Improve knowledge of anatomic and physiologic changes related to alterations of bladder blood supply

Focused Research Plans for Common Clinical Conditions

Many diseases have bladder manifestations, but several conditions affect large populations. The BRPRG has focused on a number of high-impact bladder conditions and has recommended research priorities for them. High-impact conditions include:

- Problems of the developing genitourinary tract in children

- Urologic disease in maturation and aging

- Bladder outlet obstruction

- Interstitial cystitis

- Urinary tract infections

- Urologic effects of diabetes

- Urinary incontinence

- Cancer

Problems of the Developing Genitourinary Tract in Children

Normal bladder function is a critical part of human development. Abnormal development can have a profound impact on bladder and kidney function and on psychological and social development. Abnormal development can cause the inability to control urine, resulting in intermittent wetness from urinary leakage and urinary retention; infection; pain; and, at times, kidney dysfunction and failure.

Genitourinary tract abnormalities are the most common birth abnormality. Dilatation of the urinary tract occurs in most developmental problems, and prenatal ultrasonography may identify this in as many as 1 in 500 pregnancies. Vesicoureteral reflux, one of the most common causes of kidney failure in children, occurs in an estimated 1 percent to 2 percent of newborns. In addition, at 10 years of age, as many as 5 percent of children still do not have bladder control.

With normal development, the bladder is a supple, expandable organ. Urine is transported from the kidneys to the bladder via the ureters, and the bladder serves to store urine. As humans mature, control over the bladder occurs with development, and the bladder can then be willfully emptied at socially acceptable times. Injury, disease during development, or even aging may interrupt normal development, causing problems of inadequate storage or emptying so that frequency, urgency, leakage, vesicoureteral reflux, infections, stones, or kidney deterioration may occur.

Birth defects related to the urinary tract alone or to abnormal development in other systems of the body have lifelong consequences. These defects include the following:

- Myelodysplasia (e.g., spina bifida)

- Congenital and acquired bladder outlet obstruction (e.g., posterior urethral valves, ectopic ureteroceles, dysfunctional voiding)

- Vesicoureteral reflux

- Congenital anatomic anomalies (e.g., bladder exstrophy, neurogenic bladder with imperforate anus or cloaca, and prune belly syndrome)

Complications of birth defects cause social and psychological maladjustment in addition to lifelong high medical expenses.

Research addressing developmental anomalies of the lower urinary tract is lacking. As of July 2001, only five studies of the lower urinary tract could be identified as being supported by the National Institutes of Health. Although attempts to examine the reason for abnormal bladder contractility following abnormal development are ongoing, progress in understanding even normal fetal and developmental bladder physiology is slow.

Better understanding of the developmental abnormalities will have to occur before methods to prevent these problems and their consequences can be identified.

RECOMMENDATIONS FOR GENITOURINARY TRACT PROBLEMS IN CHILDREN RESEARCH

→ Improve understanding of lower urinary tract development and dysfunction

→ Determine risk factors for abnormal urinary tract development and its consequences

→ Identify preventive measures to decrease risk

→ Develop better management and treatment

Urologic Disease in Maturation and Aging; Obstruction

In both sexes, aging appears to cause a decline in bladder contractility and an increase in involuntary contractions leading to classic lower urinary tract symptoms including nighttime voiding (nocturia) and urge incontinence. Both factors have profound effects on bladder emptying and storage. After their childbearing years, women almost universally encounter change in bladder and urethral function; however, understanding of the aging process at the cellular and molecular levels remains rudimentary. Moreover, even though the consequences of benign prostatic hyperplasia (BPH) cause problems for many men, limited effort has been directed toward prevention and treatment options.

RECOMMENDATIONS FOR MATURATION AND AGING RESEARCH

→ Examine the aging urinary tract at the cellular and molecular levels to understand the changes causing bladder dysfunction

→ Investigate and identify the molecular, cellular, gender, and potentially genetic factors that lead to dysfunction of aging

→ Develop preventive, management, and therapeutic interventions

RECOMMENDATIONS FOR BLADDER OUTLET
OBSTRUCTION RESEARCH

➡ Identify the impact of age on BPH pathophysiology
and treatment outcomes

➡ Analyze central and peripheral nervous system
contributions to voiding dysfunction and identify
related potential therapies

➡ Identify new therapeutic targets by determining
genomic and proteomic urinary tract changes
caused by obstruction

Interstitial Cystitis

Interstitial cystitis (IC) is a debilitating, chronic bladder
syndrome that causes urinary urgency and frequency
often associated with continual pelvic and bladder pain.
Although exact prevalence is unknown, it is estimated
that 700,000 to one million people have IC in this
country. The incidence in Americans has been reported
to be three times that in Europe and about the same as
the number of people who have inflammatory bowel
disease and Parkinson's disease.

Although anyone can have IC, 90 percent of sufferers
are reported to be women in their most productive years.
Fifty percent of IC patients are unable to work full-time.
In 1988, IC was estimated to cost $1.7 billion in medical
expenses and lost wages, costs that would be significantly
higher today considering rising costs and greater numbers of patients. According to a 1990 report, people on
kidney dialysis have a better quality of life than people
who have IC.

The diagnosis of IC is difficult to make. While theories
abound, there is no known cause. As a result, neither
a cure nor a consistently effective therapy is available.
Symptoms of IC may be either mistaken for a urinary
tract infection or considered to be nothing more than a
reflection of the patient's anxiety. This delays diagnosis.

Lesions of pinpoint bladder bleeding are hallmarks of
IC, but they are often seen only under general anesthesia
when the bladder is examined with a cystoscope, thus
making diagnosis difficult. Although some ongoing
research has been trying to establish the cause of IC,
none has been found. However, other avenues of research
are looking to establish conclusive diagnostic markers of
the disease that would improve diagnosis and enhance
further research on management and treatment.

RECOMMENDATIONS FOR INTERSTITIAL CYSTITIS RESEARCH

➡ Establish epidemiology and natural history of IC

➡ Identify disease markers for diagnosis and progression

➡ Conduct IC management and therapy trials

➡ Educate the public and health profession

Urinary Tract Infection

Urinary tract infections (UTIs) are common among
women, men, and children. Adult women have about a
50 percent lifetime risk of developing a UTI, and it has
been reported that by age 24, one-third of women have
had one. When they occur in special populations of risk,
including young children and the elderly, UTIs can cause
pain, severe illness, loss of kidney function, and high
blood pressure. In addition, UTIs currently account for
more than a third of the 2 million infections that occur
in hospitals each year. Most of these UTIs are secondary
to an indwelling urethral catheter. Catheter-related UTI
has been estimated to be responsible for 40 percent of
all institution-related infections. The total annual cost
of UTIs in the United States has been estimated to be
greater than $1 billion, and this estimate does not
include hospital costs.

Children are at special risk for UTIs. Approximately 3
percent of prepubertal girls and 1 percent of prepubertal
boys are diagnosed annually with UTIs. Approximately 18
percent of infants who develop a UTIs during their first

year of life experience a recurrence during subsequent months. Recurrent UTIs in infants and children are associated with significant morbidity, including impaired kidney function, end-stage renal disease, and possible complications of pregnancy. Other people at risk of developing severe complications from UTI include people with neurogenic bladders caused by diabetes or other diseases that impair the nervous system, people with catheters, pregnant women, the elderly, and people with kidney transplants.

Factors that cause or allow bacteria to attach to the skin, enter, and then ascend the urinary tract to the kidney and, at times, enter the blood stream are not well defined. Although a routine UTI often can be easily treated with antimicrobial drugs, this is not always the case. Certain bacteria have been identified that have a particular virulence for the urinary tract. These bacteria are constantly changing and becoming resistant to the antimicrobial agents currently available. For people who are at high risk of complications or who get frequent recurrent UTIs, some strides have been made to block UTI with vaccines. These vaccines are being developed and their long-term efficacy will need to be examined.

RECOMMENDATIONS FOR URINARY TRACT INFECTION RESEARCH

➡ Determine host-pathogen interactions

➡ Identify bacterial pathogenesis

➡ Identify host-cell responses

➡ Determine host susceptibility to infection and inflammation

Urologic Consequences of Diabetes Mellitus

At least 25 percent of Americans who have diabetes mellitus will develop urinary tract complications of diabetes such as urinary incontinence or retention, infection, or other lower urinary tract symptoms, but the true incidence of urinary tract dysfunction associated with diabetes is unknown. It is unknown because little attention has been focused in this area.

What is known, however, is that people with diabetes suffer from increased complications of urinary tract infections, such as kidney abscesses, papillary necrosis, and gas-forming infections of the kidney (emphysematous pyelonephritis) that may be lethal. In the United States, diabetes is probably the most common condition associated with kidney papillary necrosis, which is most likely related to a combination of diabetes and urinary tract infection.

People with diabetes also develop voiding difficulties that manifest as incontinence and urinary retention. These voiding problems are probably related to a common complication of diabetes—sensory neuropathy. In observational studies, men and women with diabetes had a 30 percent to 70 percent increased risk of urinary incontinence.

Although general research on diabetes mellitus improves our understanding of the disease, specific issues related to the urinary tract need to be examined. The pathophysiology of urinary tract dysfunction and urinary tract infection in people with diabetes is so little known that no efforts to determine risk or to predict or prevent these complicating problems have been made. In addition, almost nothing is known about the combined effect on the bladder of diabetes and prostatic enlargement, a problem that occurs in most aging men, or about the combined effects of diabetes, pregnancy, and childbirth in women.

RECOMMENDATIONS FOR DIABETIC BLADDER RESEARCH

➡ Identify and characterize changes in the diabetic bladder at the molecular and cellular level

➡ Identify markers and risk factors that predict early urinary tract involvement

➡ Examine the clinical history of disease progression with relation to gender, ethnicity, and race

➡ Perform clinical trials to identify efficacious preventive and therapeutic strategies

Urinary Incontinence

About 13 million Americans, most of them women, suffer from urinary incontinence, a problem often associated with pregnancy, childbirth, and aging. In addition, many diseases and conditions are associated with incontinence, including spinal cord injury or abnormalities, Parkinson's disease, multiple sclerosis, and diabetes. After pregnancy and childbirth, about 30 percent of women develop problems with bladder control, and almost 30 percent of all people over age 60 have some urinary leakage. In older Americans, problems with bladder control cause urgent trips to the bathroom, thus increasing the risk of falls and subsequent fractures by an estimated 20 percent to 30 percent.

Although new imaging techniques have improved our current knowledge of the anatomy of the pelvic area, the reasons for different forms of incontinence remain understudied and elusive. Different kinds of surgical operations have been developed to improve urinary incontinence in females, but few of these operations have been validated by quantitative outcome measures and few have withstood the test of time. The reasons for failure of many initially successful operations are not totally clear;

however, failure may relate to lack of understanding of the basic mechanisms of incontinence and the changes that occur with aging.

To improve the overall quality of life of Americans affected by urinary incontinence, an investment in research is needed to enhance our understanding of continence and incontinence, to identify risk factors and quantitative measures of incontinence severity, and to develop effective preventive efforts and treatment. This will require multidisciplinary investigations from basic scientists, bioengineers, and clinicians who specialize in the management, measurement, and imaging of male and female incontinence.

RECOMMENDATIONS FOR URINARY INCONTINENCE RESEARCH

➡ Develop novel techniques to measure neural, muscular, and vascular function of the bladder

➡ Identify risk factors related to childbirth and aging

➡ Improve understanding of the mechanisms of urinary incontinence

➡ Develop a national registry and tissue bank of patients suffering from urinary incontinence

Bladder Cancer

Bladder cancer is the sixth most commonly diagnosed, non-cutaneous cancer in Americans. Currently, 400,000 Americans have been estimated to have a diagnosed case of bladder cancer. These patients undergo continued surveillance examinations that are costly and invasive. For this reason, the development of new techniques for detection, prevention, chemoprevention, and treatment are imperative. Furthermore, the research community needs to investigate the basic biology of cancer in the bladder epithelium (urothelium) and develop disease models to examine abnormal cellular growth, regulation, cell-cell interaction and signaling, differentiation and control, field effect versus clonality, and urothelial alterations with age and gender to understand why this cancer has increased so rampantly and to discover markers, ways to prevent the disease, and new treatments.

Advances in imaging that make use of virtual endoscopy, contact microscopy, fluorescent cystoscopy, novel ultrasound examinations, magnetic resonance imaging (MRI), and positron emission tomography (PET) could lead to more rapid diagnosis, less invasive management, and more successful outcomes.

RECOMMENDATIONS FOR BLADDER CANCER RESEARCH

➡ Use the bladder as a model to study and treat cancer

➡ Develop and test bladder cancer preventive measures

➡ Identify new bladder cancer markers to replace current invasive bladder cancer testing

Methodologies & Technologies

Clinical Trials and Epidemiology

Methodologies such as bioinformatics, epidemiology, and advances in computer technology permit linkage of patient and disease data and allow clinical research to be performed using databases that surpass previous capabilities and capacities. These methodologies and technologies apply new rigor to clinical trials involving outcomes evaluations and neural networks. In studies of complex conditions, bioinformatics and biostatistics allow scientists to make inferences and conclusions that were previously impossible to make.

RECOMMENDATIONS FOR CLINICAL TRIALS AND EPIDEMIOLOGY RESEARCH

➡ Fund pilot studies with potential for high risk and high gain

➡ Prioritize clinical studies in which short-term gain and extramural funding are unlikely. These studies include

- Alternative therapies

- Prevention studies

- Long-term outcome studies

- Behavioral studies

- Surgical trials

➡ Develop national clinical trials and a data center with core consultation services

- Outcomes analysis

- Biostatistics

- Bioethics

- Epidemiology

➡ Establish multi-center studies to examine low-incidence, high-impact bladder problems

➡ Provide industrial partner grants to examine factors that may not be the interests of industry but can be performed simultaneously ("piggy-back" grants)

Clinical trials of bladder disease are scarce. Enormous opportunities for data gathering and for examination of best practices and management of bladder disease exist through clinical bladder trials, yet they have been under utilized and under funded in the area of bladder research.

Emerging Technologies and Pharmacology

Current advances in biotechnology have created progress in other areas of scientific endeavor at a rapid rate. All areas of bladder research and all patients with bladder-associated health problems would benefit from

- New biologic (cellular or molecular) and functional imaging techniques and genomics or proteomics techniques to identify persons at risk for bladder disease or dysfunction

- Bioengineering technology such as stem cell or gene therapy or tissue engineering techniques that allow repair, replacement, or even prevention of abnormal bladder tissue or function

As rapidly as research has progressed in proteomics and genomics, pharmacologic discovery aimed at modulating, augmenting, or blocking specific receptors has also progressed. New drug delivery systems that allow drug delivery at a specific time and place are possible, and the bladder is an ideal organ in which to deliver them.

In addition the development of new technologies for biomedicine would have a great impact on how studies of the bladder, urethra, and pelvic floor are conducted. Technologies currently in use by many researchers are usually low throughput technologies, meaning that the number of tests they can perform in a given period of time is low, a limitation that hampers the study of biologically heterogeneous disorders in humans. Another limitation involves research tools currently available for analyzing nucleic acids and proteins. These tools rely on large sample sizes, a problem when dealing with both humans and small animal models where starting material is limited.

RECOMMENDATIONS FOR EMERGING TECHNOLOGIES AND PHARMACOLOGY RESEARCH

→ Develop tissue and bladder renewal and replacement techniques using stem cell and tissue engineering technology

→ Develop minimally invasive diagnostic techniques for the lower urinary tract using micro-engineering and biomechanical technology to perform functional bladder imaging, urodynamics, and biomechanical assessment

→ Establish a research infrastructure focused on the bladder that includes core facilities to harness genomic (and microarray), proteomic, and bioinformatics technology

→ Support drug development and delivery systems that affect the following:

- Sensory pathways

- Micturition through the nervous system

- Muscular activity

- Blood flow

- Connective tissue

- Gene therapy

Resource and Infrastructure Needs

At this time in medicine, clinical research is severely challenged. Clinical investigators have less time for clinical research because of the increasing complexities involved in performing their day-to-day patient care activities. Clinical trials are often inadequately funded. Clinical research is expensive, and human research is highly regulated requiring high degrees of organization and support. Many bladder diseases have a long natural history, and outcomes trials must be undertaken over many years, facts that make clinical research even more complicated.

The BRPRG has concluded that current clinical research on the lower urinary tract lags behind many other disease areas because of inadequate prior funding. Building an effective program in bladder research requires not only financial support, but also an underlying infrastructure. New requests for applications (RFAs) are needed to address the listed research priorities. Efficient and effective clinical research programs are needed that not only allow recruitment of high-risk patients, minority patients, and special groups, but also provide long-term follow up. These programs must have a high regard for patient health and safety. To achieve this, a stable well-supported infrastructure of professionals who are knowledgeable in research methodology, outcomes evaluations, biostatistics, data analyses, and epidemiology is required. These resources in different forms need to be available at targeted local, regional, and national sites to assess and perform clinical research.

Because of the paucity of bladder research, the BRPRG recommends that the number of investigators interested in bladder research be increased by efforts to attract established investigators into the field and to train new investigators. The BRPRG recommends that this be achieved by prioritizing RFAs of collaborative research and by establishing a mechanism for program and proposal review and evaluation that is specific to the lower urinary tract. The BRPRG also recommends that establishment of a planning group for implementing these recommendations be considered at the national level.

The future of United States bladder research needs to be created today. This can be effectively accomplished by creating an infrastructure and by recruiting, training, and retaining investigators.

RECOMMENDATIONS FOR RESOURCE AND INFRASTRUCTURE NEEDS

➡ Increase the investigator workforce as follows:

- Train new investigators

- Attract established investigators into the field

➡ Create new bladder multidisciplinary research and training programs

➡ Create national resource centers

➡ Support data and tissue banks for bladder research

➡ Provide incentives for NIH-academic-industrial research initiatives

➡ Establish NIH bladder planning and review panels

Conclusion

The BRPRG has reviewed the bladder research effort funded by the federal government and has found this portfolio to be deficient both in total and in proportionate funding when compared with other organs and major disease areas that affect the human condition to a similar degree.

The United States has a large population that is affected by bladder diseases and conditions, and many of these problems have been neglected to a large part because of poor education of the public and health professionals and because of the social stigma attached to urinary processes. Social stigma has prevented many from speaking out about these problems and has undoubtedly limited the number of public advocacy groups that have formed. In addition, some people with these conditions—children, the elderly, and people with neurological impairments—are unable to be advocates.

The United States has been a leader in biomedical research, and it can play a major role in the effort to improve the lives of people with bladder-impairing conditions.

To implement the recommendations in this report, the Executive Committee of the BRPRG asks the National Institute of Diabetes and Digestive and Kidney Diseases and other institutes and centers of the National Institutes of Health (NIH) to increase bladder research funding over a seven-year period. Other institutes and programs of the NIH might also contribute to this effort by recognizing the bladder component of many diseases that are already being studied. Substantial increases in funding will allow bladder research levels to become commensurate with other important areas of human problems.

With the continually increasing life expectancy of the American public, bladder conditions will have a rising impact on the United States in social and economic proportions. An investment in research funding at this time has the potential to improve the quality of life of the American people and to dramatically decrease the emotional, psychological, societal, and financial burden of bladder diseases.

SECTION A BASIC SCIENCE OF THE LOWER URINARY TRACT

Although it appears to be a simple storage organ, the bladder is physiologically more complex than previously thought. Recent studies have revealed exquisitely timed biochemical interactions occurring between cells in the bladder's various tissue layers and the peripheral and central nervous systems that synchronize the storing and releasing of urine. These interactions, when normal, create a seamless chain of events that is often taken for granted by healthy people. However, a disturbance in one part of this intricate system can affect other parts, leading to dysfunction, disease, and poor quality of life.

The lower urinary tract comprises the bladder, the ureters, the bladder outlet (vesical neck and urethra), and the sphincter muscle. Predominantly a muscular organ, the bladder stores and empties urine.

Urine flows from the kidneys through two ureters, which are long tubes inserted into the bladder, a balloon-like structure made of a thin layer of smooth (visceral) muscle. The bladder stores the urine, stretching as it fills. A sphincter muscle located where the bladder opens into the urethra prevents urine from leaking. This circular, striated (skeletal) muscle or sphincter is in a state of contraction until it receives a message from the brain to relax.

The storage capacity of the bladder is about 10 to 20 ounces of urine. When the bladder has about half its capacity, nerves send signals to the brain that the bladder is getting full. During voiding, the sphincter relaxes, the bladder muscle (detrusor) contracts, and urine is voluntarily discharged into the urethra, the canal through which urine is expelled from the body.

Dramatic changes occur in the lower urinary tract during a person's lifetime. In the fetus, the bladder initially serves as a conduit that transmits urine from the ureter and dispels it through the urachus, the fetal urinary canal located between the bladder and the umbilicus, into the amniotic fluid. Eventually, the bladder expands and becomes a prototype storage organ in the fetus. Later in fetal development and in the newborn, the bladder develops reflex activity controlled by the central nervous system. At first, reflex emptying is inefficient, but it becomes more efficient as the nervous system matures and is able to coordinate the functions of the urethra and urethral sphincter with those of the bladder.

During reflex voiding, the detrusor muscle and the epithelium of the bladder send a message that the bladder is full over afferent (ingoing) pathways into the spinal cord. The spinal cord transmits this information to a switching circuit in the brain stem that automatically turns on and relays the information back through the spinal cord and efferent (outgoing) nerves to the bladder, which then empties. Eventually the cerebral cortex takes control over the brain stem.

During early childhood, the bladder develops as a sensory organ. Sensation is a function that must develop in children for them to realize the bladder is full. When this occurs, voluntary control of urination or voiding can be achieved. The cerebral cortex allows voluntary control, that is, the system can be turned on and off at will. Normal voiding depends on good coordination between the brain and the spinal cord.

The bladder is composed of smooth muscle, the type of muscle that is found in most organs of the body; epithelium; connective tissue; nerves; and blood vessels. Complex biochemical interactions that are still being discovered occur among these structures. Therefore, this finely tuned system is not always in a steady state during a person's lifetime, as research and life experiences have revealed. Diseases and conditions such as multiple sclerosis and stroke, infection, hereditary factors, diabetes, injury to the peripheral and central nervous systems, and aging, to name a few, can reverse this development process.

CHAPTER 1

UROTHELIUM

Basic Science of the Lower Urinary Tract

DID YOU KNOW?

→ The urothelium—epithelial tissue lining the inner surface of the lower urinary tract—functions as a barrier to micro-organisms and toxins and may also act as a sensory organ.

→ Practically every major disease of the bladder, including cancer, interstitial cystitis, and infection, involves the urothelium.

→ The urothelium holds great potential for research studies because it is readily accessible.

Summary and Recommendations

The inner surface of the urinary tract is lined with epithelial tissue or urothelium, which functions as a barrier to bacteria, environmental carcinogens, toxins, and the highly variable waste products in urine. Practically every major disease of the bladder, including cancer, infection, inflammation, and developmental anomalies, involves the urothelium.

Studies of the urothelium hold great potential for making an impact on the treatment of not only urologic diseases, but also diseases in other areas of the body. The Bladder Research Progress Review Group has made the following recommendations (in order of priority) for research on lower urinary tract urothelium:

➡ **Determine how normal urothelium develops and performs its unique biological functions by investigating the following:**

- Synthesis, assembly, and function of urothelial cell differentiation products

- Influence of cell-cell interactions and other extracellular signals on urothelial biology

- Molecular bases of the urothelium's permeability barrier function

- Secretion of urinary proteins, including growth factors

- Possible urothelial involvement in the function of nerve cells

- Identification of additional urothelial differentiation markers (factors by which a cell or molecule can be recognized and identified) using cDNA microarray and tissue array technologies

→ **Determine how the urothelium develops pathology in response to disease-causing stimuli by identifying**

- Interactions between uropathogenic bacteria, the urothelium, and the mechanisms of recurrent UTI

- Altered oncogenes (genes that encode proteins involved in cell growth and regulation that when mutated can cause abnormal cell growth) and other genetic mutation

- Urine components, including carcinogenes and tumor-promoting agents, toxins, and growth-modulating factors

- Abnormal urothelial gene expression patterns by using cDNA microarray and tissue array technologies

→ **Develop shared resources for urothelial research as follows:**

- Develop a "urochip," a cDNA microarray chip specific to urologic and bladder genes

- Expand and support new technology, including proteomics and tissue arrays

- Develop bioinformatics to analyze the high throughput data (data that can be generated efficiently in a few tests in a relatively short time)

- Develop multi-institutional tissue banks, tissue registries, and transgenic repositories

- Increase funding to support training grants and shared core facilities

→ **Determine the differences in structure and function of urothelial cells from different regions of the urinary tract.** This will provide critical baseline information for all future studies on urothelial biology and diseases.

→ **Identify the mesenchymal signals that direct the differentiation pathways of urothelial cells.** The striking plasticity of adult urothelium, which can differentiate into prostate-, colon- and seminal-vesicle-like structures in response to mesenchymal signals, provides unique opportunities to better understand mesenchymal-urothelial interaction and urothelial differentiation.

→ **Identify the roles of urinary markers in the pathogenesis of interstitial cystitis (IC).** At least six urine markers have been shown in blinded studies to be significantly different between IC patients and controls. These differences may provide clues to the pathogenetic mechanism for this poorly understood bladder disorder.

→ **Determine the effects of age and gender on urothelial structure and function.**

→ **Delineate the effects of mechanical stretching on urothelial growth and apical surface area expansion, and determine the molecular bases for such regulation.**

→ **Elucidate the structure and function of the urothelial glycocalyx, a filamentous coating on the apical surface of certain bladder urothelial cells, or glycosoaminoglycan (GAG), a protein-polysaccharide complex lining the apical surface of bladder urothelial cells, in normal urothelial biology and in interstitial cystitis.**

→ **Develop and characterize additional *in vitro* (test tube) models of urothelial growth and differentiation using both human and other mammalian urothelial cells for studying urothelial-mesenchymal interactions and their roles in disease processes.**

→ **Develop and characterize additional novel animal models for urothelial diseases.**

Background

The urothelium is the major tissue lining the surface of almost the entire urinary tract. Recent research has indicated that the urothelium functions somewhat like the nervous system; that is, urothelial cells express receptors and release transmitters such as nitric oxide and adenosine triphosphate (ATP). Thus, urothelial cells appear to play a role in normal bladder sensation. What is not known, however, is whether the urothelium functions as a sensory organ throughout the different stages of development.

The urothelium also functions as a barrier to bacteria, environmental carcinogens, toxins, and the highly variable waste products in urine. Consequently, practically every major disease of the bladder involves the urothelium. The following are just a few:

➡ **Urothelial cancer**—Ninety-five percent of all bladder cancer is urothelial cancer, which annually affects 56,000 Americans and is the fifth most commonly diagnosed non-skin malignancy in this country.

➡ **Urinary tract infection**—Urinary tract infection, or UTI as it is commonly referred to, affects both sexes, but significantly more women than men. Every year an estimated 7 million cases of uncomplicated UTI occur in the United States. Bacteria known as type 1-fimbriated or piliated *Escherichia coli* cause more than 90 percent of the cases. These bacteria attach to urothelial cell surface receptors before invading the urinary tract. Without such initial binding to the urothelium, the bacteria would be removed by urination and no infection could occur. Invasion of type 1-piliated *E. coli* into the kidney may be responsible for more than 250,000 cases of kidney infection (pyelonephritis). The emergence of bacteria resistant to antibiotics presents a serious health problem.

➡ **Interstitial cystitis**—Known as the "painful bladder syndrome," interstitial cystitis is an extremely debilitating condition affecting an estimated 700,000 to 1 million people in the United States, mostly females. Defects in the urothelium are thought to play a major role in this problem.

➡ **Vesicoureteral reflux**—A hereditary problem affecting almost 1 percent to 2 percent of all children, vesicoureteral reflux can cause serious kidney damage even before a child is born and is one of the leading causes of kidney failure in children.

Studies of the urothelium hold great potential for making an impact on the treatment of not only urologic diseases, but also diseases in other areas. Urothelium is both readily accessible to routine examination and particularly plastic in terms of developmental potential. Thus, it provides unique opportunities for a better understanding of (1) interactions between the mesenchyme and urothelium and (2) determination of tissue fate during embryonic development.

In addition, the urothelium exhibits intriguing biological properties, including colonization of the bladder by multiple tumors in separate locations (the "field effect"); this phenomenon occurs despite the entire urothelium being bathed in and exposed to the same urine environment. Finally, normal and diseased human urothelial cells are readily available for study. For these reasons, urothelial research has the potential for revealing basic biologic principles that are of value to all fields of scientific inquiry.

Research Advances and Opportunities

Reducing the morbidity and mortality of widespread debilitating conditions of the lower urinary tract will depend on future research projects that focus on achieving a better understanding of the following:

- Differences in the structure of urothelial cells from different regions of the urinary tract

- Regulation of urothelial growth and differentiation

- Cellular and molecular bases of urothelial diseases

- Differences in the function of urothelial cells

Differences in Structure of Urothelial Cells

Urothelial cells from the renal pelvis, ureter, bladder, and proximal urethra traditionally have been thought to be the same cell types. However, subtle, but potentially important, gender- or age-related urothelial differences exist.

Some recent studies suggest that urothelial cells may be more heterogeneous than previously thought. Urothelial cells from the ureters, kidneys, and trigone region of the bladder (the area of the bladder that forms a triangle between the insertion of the two ureters and the point where the urethra begins) are thought to be derived from the embryonic mesoderm, while urothelial cells of the urethra and the bladder wall, excluding the trigone, are derived from the embryonic endoderm.

Tissue recombination studies indicate that urothelial cells from different regions of the lower urinary tract can give rise to various types of urothelial cells when signaled by various embryonic mesenchyme. Thus, the endoderm-derived bladder urothelium gives rise to prostate tissue in response to embryonic urogenital or seminal vesicle mesenchyme, while the mesoderm-derived ureter urothelium gives rise to seminal vesicle cells. Taken together, these data raise the intriguing possibility that significant cellular, structural, and functional differences may exist among the urothelial cells of different regions of the urinary tract. This concept has significant implications in the biology and pathogenesis of urothelial diseases.

Urothelial Differentiation Markers and Diseases

Characterization of genes differentially expressed in urothelial cells is an important step towards a better understanding of urothelial structure and function. Recently, a group of uroplakins—integral membrane proteins—has been identified as the major differentiation (specialization) product of mammalian urothelial cells. Studies of uroplakins have led to a better understanding of several important bladder diseases and conditions, including urinary tract infection, bladder cancer formation, and vesicoureteral reflux, a congenital anomaly.

For example, uroplakin Ia is a receptor for type 1-piliated *Escherichia coli*, a bacterium involved in recurrent UTIs and antibiotic resistance. The binding of type 1-piliated *E. coli* to uroplakin receptors is facilitated by the bacteria's filamentous projections called pili or fimbriae. Bacterial attachment can result in at least two effects, one leading to programmed cell death (apoptosis) and shedding (exfoliation) of urothelial cells, possibly as a way of host self-defense, and the other leading to bacterial invasion into urothelial cells and propagation. Understanding bacterial invasion is important for developing better treatments for antibiotic resistance and infection relapse. A vaccine that blocks type 1-piliated *E. coli* from attaching to urothelial cells is being developed and has shown promising results in animal studies and human trials.

Studies of the promoter of the uroplakin II gene helped define the roles of specific oncogenes in bladder cancer. Oncogenes are genes normally responsible for making proteins involved in regulating cell growth. However, when these genes are mutated or abnormally activated, they can make altered proteins that lead to uncontrolled cell growth or tumor formation. For example, the oncogene, SV40T, when directed by the uroplakin II promoter to express in the bladder urothelium resulted in the formation of localized bladder cancer and later, full-blown transitional cell cancer. In contrast, H-RAS, an oncogene frequently activated in melanoma and in cancer of the colon, lung, and pancreas, led to the formation of a papillary tumor. This provided strong evidence supporting the two-pathway hypothesis of bladder tumor development.

Another recent study has established that the Tamm-Horsfall protein, a mucoprotein contained in the mucus urothelial cells of the bladder and the most abundant protein in human urine, is the major defense factor for preventing type 1-piliated *E. coli* from adhering to the uroplakin receptors on urothelial cells in the bladder.

Finally, the genetic ablation of the uroplakin III gene in mice has resulted in the formation of grossly abnormal superficial (umbrella) urothelial cells, which are functionally deficient because they form an inferior permeability barrier, a condition that would increase susceptibility to toxins and possibly uropathogenic microorganisms. In addition, the mice suffered from vesicoureteral reflux, the retrograde flow of urine from the bladder into the ureters and kidneys. This surprising finding is important because it suggests that genetic defects causing urothelial abnormalities can result in reflux, an important pediatric urologic problem that can have a significant effect on families because 30 percent of siblings of children with known reflux will have the disorder as well.

It has also been suggested that a glycosaminoglycan (GAG) layer (a protein-polysaccharide complex) lining the apical surface of bladder urothelial cells inhibits bacterial adherence and contributes to the urothelium's function as a barrier to microorganisms and toxins. The composition and function of GAG has been the subject of much discussion and needs to be studied further.

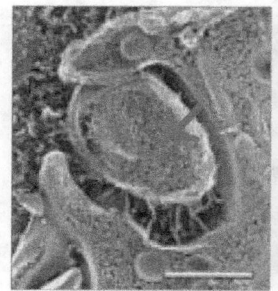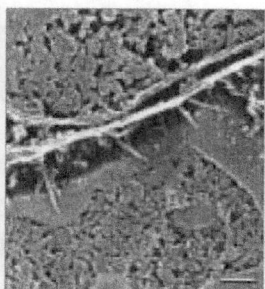

Two hours after infection, a type 1 piliated *Escherichia coli* bacterium (left) adheres to epithelial cells on the bladder wall of a mouse. The bacterium uses pili (right) to bind to uroplakin Ia receptors in the epithelial cells. (Photo Credit: Matthew A. Mulvey, Yolanda S. Lopez-Boado, Carole L. Wilson, Robyn Roth, William C. Parks, John Heuser, and Scott J. Hultgren. Adapted from Science, 282:1494-97. Copyright 1998, the American Association for the Advancement of Science.)

Regulation of Urothelial Cell Growth and Differentiation

Abnormal urothelial cell growth appears to be related to several important bladder diseases, including cancer and interstitial cystitis; therefore, determining the roles of the factors that stimulate or inhibit cell growth in the urothelium is of great importance.

Recent data indicate that human urothelial cells synthesize many growth factors. Some of these factors are implicated in the regulation of urothelial cell growth and differentiation. Data on these factors may be relevant to interstitial cystitis, which features thinning and sometimes ulceration of the urothelium.

Studies have recently identified two novel growth-modulating factors that are both synthesized and secreted into the urine by the urothelial cells of persons with interstitial cystitis. Those growth-modulating factors are

- A small-sized growth-inhibiting factor that may have important implications as a diagnostic tool

- A small-sized urine factor that can cause the programmed cell death (apoptosis) of urothelial cells

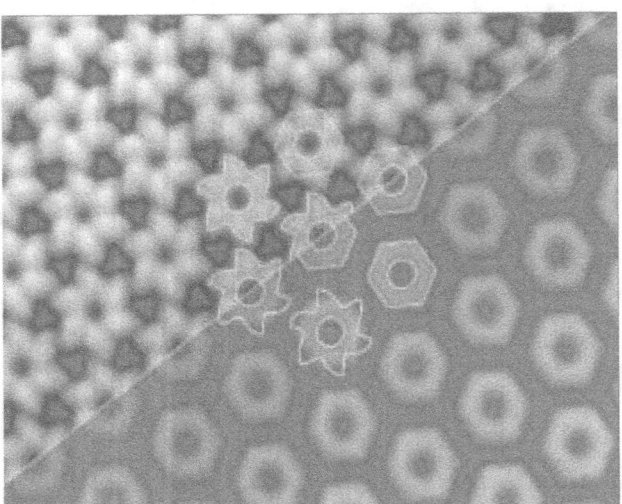

Uroplakin Ia, the urothelial receptor for bacterial adhesin FimH, is localized on the six inner domains of the 16 nm urothelial plaque particle. In this atomic force microscopy image, mouse and bovine plaques are visualized. The averaged images of the luminal (upper left half) and the cytoplasmic (lower right half) surfaces of bovine and mouse urothelial plaques, respectively, display propeller-shaped 16 nm AUM particles on the luminal surface and ~14nm diameter, circular protrusions on the cytoplasmic surface. (*Photo Credit: Guangwei Min, Martin Stolz, Ge Zhou, Fengxia Liang, Peter Sebbel, Danial Stoffler, Rudi Glockshuber, Tung-Tien Sun, Ueli Aebi, Xiang-Peng Kong. The Journal of Molecular Biology. 317:967-706. Copyright* 2002. Elsevier Science.)

Further studies of these factors, which occur mainly in persons with interstitial cystitis, may lead to an improved understanding of the pathogenesis and novel treatment of this disease.

Another interesting recent finding indicates that mechanical stretch can influence growth factor production by the bladder's smooth muscle cells. This process could play a role in both the excessive growth of bladder muscle (hypertrophy) present in many bladder diseases and in the regulation of urothelial growth.

Novel Urothelial Cell Functions

Although the urothelium has been traditionally thought of as a permeability barrier, recent studies indicate that it is functionally versatile. These studies have discovered that (1) the urothelium can secrete a variety of proteins into the urine in addition to certain growth factors and (2) activation of urothelial cells by mechanical, chemical, or noxious stimuli results in the release of neurotransmitters such as nitric oxide and adenosine triphosphate (ATP), which may stimulate adjacent nerves.

- **Secretion of proteins and growth factors.** The urothelium can secrete a variety of proteins into the urine in addition to certain growth factors. This activity has a potentially practical application; the promoter of the uroplakin gene in transgenic mice (mice that have had a gene transplant in which new DNA was introduced into their germ cells by injection into the nucleus of the ovum) could be used to drive the urothelial production and secretion of pharmaceutically important human recombinant proteins such as human growth factors.

- **Release of neurotransmitters.** Activation of urothelial cells by mechanical, chemical, or noxious stimuli results in the release of neurotransmitters such as nitric oxide and adenosine triphosphate (ATP), which may stimulate adjacent nerves. In addition, urothelial cells exhibit functional capsaicin receptors, proteins that are located in nerves that detect certain types of pain. These observations raise the possibility that urothelial cells may communicate with nerve receptors that convey stimuli to the central nervous system via chemical signaling between cells, thereby participating in normal bladder sensation. Because abnormal interactions between the urothelium and nerve cells could play a role in painful bladder disorders such as interstitial cystitis, these new findings suggest that urothelium can function in several new ways, and that defects in these processes could play a role in certain bladder disorders.

Mechanisms of Urothelial Permeability Barrier Function

Because the composition of urine differs sharply from that of blood, the urothelium must block the passage of many molecules that normally pass freely across biological membranes. These molecules include water, urea, and ammonia. As a result, the urothelium has evolved as the most effective permeability barrier known to exist in mammals. This is attributed to both the tight junctions interconnecting the superficial urothelial cells (umbrella cells) and the highly specialized urothelial apical surface membranes.

Recent studies have indicated that both membrane lipids and proteins contribute to the permeability barrier function. The availability of *in vitro* (test tube) and *in vivo* (animal) model systems opens new avenues for further studies on the roles of specific proteins and lipids in urothelial barrier function. *In vitro* systems can also be useful for studying the effects of antibiotics and certain proteins secreted by eosinophils—a type of white blood cell associated with inflammation—on urothelial barrier function. These proteins may play a role in disease states.

Research Requirements

Workforce

Training grants should be available to prepare young investigators for a career in bladder research. In addition, special grants designed to attract established investigators to bladder research will be highly desirable.

Infrastructure

Establishment of multi-center programs would aid research projects that require the recruitment of large patient populations, such as projects for bladder cancer or vesicoureteral reflux.

Shared Resources

Resources that can be shared by all investigators would facilitate and expedite research studies. These resources are as follows:

- **Tissue banks.** A major impediment to urothelial research has been the lack of well-controlled clinical specimens. A tissue bank of normal and diseased human bladder biopsy and urine specimens will be tremendously helpful to the urothelial research community.

- **Bladder-specific microarray chips.** Commercial microarray chips usually do not contain some of the genes of unique interest to bladder research, such as urothelial-specific genes. The National Institutes of Health (NIH) should consider the possibility of funding the development of such special reagents.

- **Depository of transgenic and knockout mouse embryos.** Many transgenic mouse lines, potentially useful for bladder research, are lost when they become too expensive for individual laboratories to maintain or to store as frozen embryos. A depository of frozen embryos, funded by the NIH, will alleviate the waste of these potentially valuable resources. A website at NIH listing the available shared resources such as these frozen embryos would be useful.

- **Exploratory research technologies.** Many currently available technologies, such as cDNA microarrays, subtraction libraries, gene ablation techniques, and the genomic project, are mainly exploratory in nature (as opposed to hypothesis-driven). These technologies have generated extremely useful information and surprising new insights into a variety of human diseases. The use of such technologies is grossly under-funded in the urothelial field, and their use needs to be encouraged by the National Institute of Diabetes and Digestive and Kidney Diseases (NIDDK). Requests for Application (RFAs) in these areas would be highly desirable.

Randy Hunter

Bladder Cancer, Cystectomy, Urinary Diversion

In October 2000, Randy Hunter noticed blood in his urine. When it didn't go away after a few days, he went to his primary care physician, who thought it might be a bladder infection and treated him with a course of antibiotics. The bleeding continued, however, and Hunter's doctor referred him to a urologist who performed a cystoscopy, a procedure that uses a fiberoptic scope to view the inside of the bladder. During that procedure, a tumor was discovered, and it was resected along with a portion of the bladder muscle. A biopsy revealed that Hunter, age 44, had invasive bladder cancer.

"It surprised both my doctor and me because of my relatively young age at the time and because I was not a smoker and didn't drink alcohol excessively," Hunter says. He also notes that he had never lived in rural areas where there are wells that could be contaminated with carcinogens or in areas with known industrial toxins in the environment. Hunter also puzzles over the fact that he had no symptoms before the blood appeared, although in retrospect, he did have a problem sitting through the duration of his sons' soccer games.

A week and a half after cancer was diagnosed, Hunter's bladder, prostate gland, and surrounding lymph nodes were removed, and a urinary diversion was performed. A urinary diversion involves connecting the ureters to a portion of the small intestine, usually the ileum or jejunum, which is looped off and used as reservoir for urine. While the ureters are inserted into one end of the loop, the other end is fashioned into a stoma and is brought out through the skin.

In a traditional urinary diversion such as an ileostomy, a plastic bag is sealed to the skin around the stoma, and urine collects in the bag. However, Hunter's surgeon performed a relatively new procedure called a continent urinary diversion, which means that Hunter can retain urine in the intestinal reservoir and use intermittent catheterization to drain it. Patients who have this procedure do not have to wear a bag.

In the continent urinary diversion, the surgeon uses a portion of the bowel where the small intestine joins the large intestine. This area has a natural valve that can be incorporated into the stoma, allowing the stoma to close until a catheter is inserted and the urine is drained. The stoma is usually located near the navel. Patients who have a urinary diversion can remain continent between catheterizations.

After two weeks in the hospital, "basically getting my strength back and dealing with the hoses coming out of me," Hunter was discharged with a temporary urinary catheter and two abdominal drains. "It was a little rough for a while," he says.

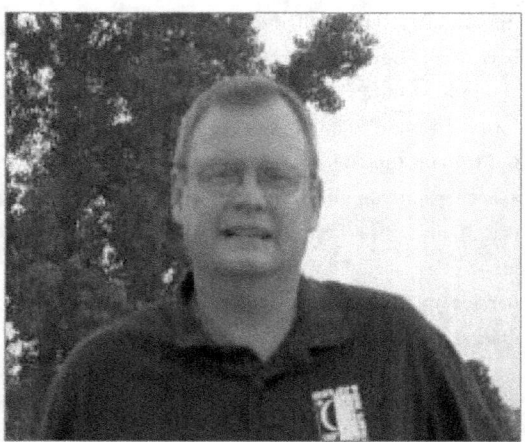

During his first few weeks at home, Hunter had to learn to change his bandages and flush the catheter so that it wouldn't become clogged from the mucous that is normally manufactured by the intestinal mucosa.

"The first few times it was a little scary," says Hunter, who had visiting nurses helping him, "but once I learned the routine and learned to recognize when it was becoming clogged, I got used to it." The routine became easier after the catheter and drains were removed in the third week after surgery.

At first, Hunter catheterized himself intermittently every three hours, but gradually moved up to four as his intestinal pouch stretched. "You think that three hours is not a problem, but you have to plan your life so that you can be near a bathroom," Hunter explains. "Some public restrooms aren't that convenient or clean."

Wherever he goes, Hunter carries with him disposable catheters and lubricating gel. Catheterization must be as clean as possible to avoid infection. Although he can now drain the catheter directly into the toilet, in the first few weeks of this routine, he had to measure the urine to be sure that the reservoir was draining properly. To do this, he had to carry a container as well.

In addition to catheterizing himself periodically, Hunter also has to irrigate the reservoir by flushing it with saline solution. This is to ensure that the reservoir and stoma are not clogged by mucous. He also drinks a lot of fluid to dilute the urine and mucous.

When Hunter returned to his job as an information technology specialist, he was worried that he wouldn't remember to catheterize himself and the reservoir would leak, so he set his watch alarm, something that aroused the curiosity of his co-workers. Now, he is able to sense when his "bladder" is full. He can even sleep through the night without waking up to drain it.

Eighteen months after surgery, Hunter visits his urologist and oncologist every three to four months for a physical exam and blood work, and a CT scan is done every other visit. Hunter is able to play tennis with his twin sons, who are 17, and take his 13-year-old daughter to her activities. He has also played some golf. Last April he and his wife went on a cruise, and he went swimming for the first time since his surgery. He has also become involved with the American Cancer Society's Relay for Life and is serving on the organizing committee this year.

Hunter feels fortunate that his cancer had not spread to the lymph nodes and that he did not need chemotherapy or radiation. He remains puzzled, however, about why he developed bladder cancer in the first place. He would like research to find out why. He would also like to educate people about the signs and symptoms of bladder cancer, how to prevent it, and the types of treatment that are available for it.

"Every day I'm reminded of what I went through. I see the scar and the stoma in the mirror," he says. "I want others to not have to go through this."

CHAPTER 2

CONNECTIVE TISSUE AND MATRIX

Basic Science of the Lower Urinary Tract

DID YOU KNOW?

→ Significant alterations in connective tissue of the lower urinary tract occur in pelvic organ prolapse, diabetes, incontinence, interstitial cystitis, nervous system diseases, and obstruction.

→ Connective tissue serves as a scaffold for cells and as a repository for growth factors, cytokines (proteins that regulate the intensity and duration of the immune response), and inflammatory factors.

→ Reciprocal cell signaling pathways in connective tissue are important during development, wound healing, and disease progression, but they are incompletely understood.

Summary and Recommendations

Despite the biological and medical importance of connective tissue, little is known about the chemical, physical, and mechanical characterization of this tissue and how it may become altered during development and disease or as a result of normal aging, childbirth, hormonal deprivation, and mechanical deformation or stretch. Little is also known about the potential risk factors for disease or protective factors that are related to connective tissue.

After an extensive review of past and current research on connective tissue of the bladder, the Bladder Research Progress Review Group made the following suggestions:

➡ **Develop better methods to image the bladder, preferably using non- or minimally destructive approaches**

➡ **Develop a rapid method to map the complete bladder wall fiber structure**
The major stress bearing fibers of the bladder wall (smooth muscle and collagen fibers) can withstand high tensile force but have low torsional and flexural stiffness. Thus, identifying the directions in which the tissue is able to withstand the greatest tensile stresses will identify the directions in which the fibers are oriented. Fiber orientation leads to an understanding and predictability of the mechanical properties of the tissue. Although available microscopic techniques can provide quantitative information on fiber structure, this information is by definition highly localized, making it difficult to quantify larger scale fiber structural features.

➡ **Develop a method of auto identification and segmentation from imaging data to streamline the processing of collagen, smooth muscle, cellular material, vasculature, and elastin**

➡ **Convert structural information into databases suitable for immediate use (e.g., bioinformatics and computational biomechanics applications)**

- What are the physical limits on the interactions between epithelium and other layers within the bladder wall?

- Is communication based upon cell-cell contact, diffusion of materials between cells or systemic circulation, or a combination of any of these?

Background

Connective tissue is the material between the cells of the body that gives various tissues form and strength. This composite of structural macromolecules or extracellular matrix is also involved in delivering nutrients to the tissues and in the special functioning of certain tissues. Connective tissue also connects and supports other tissues of the body, and, with few exceptions, is highly vascular. It differs from many other types of tissue because it contains relatively few cellular elements and abundant non-cellular material.

Structure and Function in the Urinary Tract

Connective tissue connects the various layers of tissues lining the urinary tract. Nerves, blood vessels, and lymph vessels also lie within its supporting structure.

In the lower urinary tract, connective tissue connects the layers of the mucous membrane to each other and to underlying parts. The mucous membrane of the urinary tract is continuous with the reproductive system in both males and females.

Connective tissue is composed of cells separated from one another by a semi-fluid ground substance composed of fibrillar proteoglycans and tissue fluid. This extracellular compartment delivers supplies from the blood to the cells and carries cellular waste products back to the blood and lymph. The matrix contains an irregular network of collagenous bundles and elastic fibers, the principal structural features of connective tissue. The collagenous bundles are composed of collagen molecules that are members of a family of structural proteins.

Collagen bundles contain many covalently cross-linked fibers that provide great tensile strength but not flexibility. In the bladder, collagen fibrils form a sheath around bundles of muscle fibrils and connect them. The elastic fibers of connective tissue contain a protein called elastin.

Other cells also lie within the extracellular matrix; these cells include plasma cells, macrophages, mast cells, and blood cells. Macrophages and mast cells perform immune system activities. Macrophages ingest and digest other cells, such as bacteria and foreign particles, and are involved in producing antibodies; mast cells produce heparin, histamine, and other proteolytic enzymes and are involved in immediate hypersensitivity reactions to perceived foreign substances. Mast cells may also play a role in the maintenance of the matrix.

Fibers found in the matrix interact with a variety of other proteins. The quantity and arrangement of these components have an impact on the non-cellular matrix; therefore, characterization of the matrix could provide important information about the passive properties of the bladder wall, ureters, and pelvic floor.

Of equal importance are the interactions that occur between the cells residing within connective tissues and the structural macromolecules themselves. Connective tissues can serve as a scaffold for cells and as a repository for growth factors, cytokines (hormone-like proteins that regulate the immune response), inflammatory factors, and factors that support or prevent the growth of blood vessels. As these materials act on the cells residing within connective tissues, the cells in turn may express altered phenotypes (forms) whose secreted products change the composition of connective tissue. These alterations can compromise the structural integrity and strength of connective tissue, thereby altering its physiologic function.

The dynamic nature of reciprocal cell signaling pathways is incompletely understood; however, these processes are important during development, wound healing, and disease progression.

Bladder Muscle and Connective Tissue

The normal, unstretched bladder has muscle bundles called fascicles, which are of varying sizes, lengths, and orientation. The fascicles run as geodesic lines around the bladder, sometimes leaving discontinuities. A collagen sheet surrounds each muscle fascicle, and wavy collagen bundles connect the muscle fascicles to each other. Each collagen bundle is in a helical coil that lengthens and thins during distention of the intact bladder.

Elastin has been found on the surface of muscle fascicles as well as within them. Because they are bundled and surrounded by collagen and elastin layers, the muscle fascicles can move independently and contract freely. In addition, the bundled structure allows for large stretches to occur in the bladder wall.

Dysfunctional Connective Tissue in the Bladder

The status of connective tissue in the lower urinary tract affects its physiologic function. It also affects other tissues that are structurally associated with connective tissue. Although connective tissue is passive, that is, it does not require metabolic energy for its function, connective tissue forms the structural and architectural framework upon which tissue integrity and tensile strength are based. Diseases and conditions such as pelvic organ prolapse, diabetes, interstitial cystitis, neuropathic bladder, and obstruction of the lower urinary tract in men secondary to benign prostatic hyperplasia (BPH) or prostate cancer are all characterized by significant alterations in connective tissue.

Despite the biological and medical importance of connective tissue, little is known about the chemical, physical, and mechanical characterization of this tissue and how it may become altered during development and disease, or as a result of normal aging, childbirth, hormonal deprivation, and mechanical deformation, that is, stretch or compression. Little is known about the potential risk factors or protective factors that are related to connective tissue.

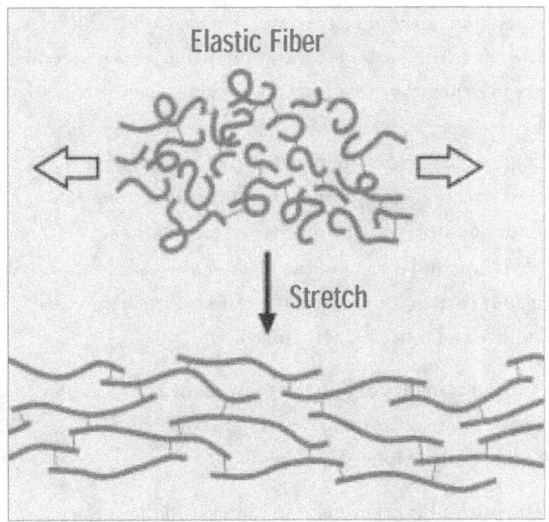

An illustration of the arrangement of elastic fibers of connective tissue at rest and during stretching. (*Courtesy of Charles Curry, PA-C, University of Florida Physician Assistant Program.*)

Connective tissue diseases or their pathologies are broadly interpreted to include deterioration of the fundamentally passive mechanical and structural characteristics of tissues that contain connective tissue. Weakened connective tissue, whatever the cause, most likely plays a role in incontinence. An example is the long-established association of urinary incontinence with menopause. This association strongly suggests that estrogen loss contributes to connective tissue deterioration, perhaps by decreasing the total collagen content in tissues.

Incontinence is a clinical symptom of altered connective tissue. It is caused by increased laxity of the pelvic floor, the sphincter muscle of the urethra, and associated structures and also by altered storage properties of the bladder. These alterations can occur during vaginal delivery or because of hysterectomy and subsequent pelvic organ prolapse.

Alterations in connective tissue can also affect children. Obstructive disorders of the lower urinary tract, secondary to either physical obstruction or obstruction caused by nervous system diseases, can be present and cause changes in bladder architecture that involve fibrosis, the formation of abnormal amounts of collagenous fiber bundles in the connective tissue matrix of the bladder wall. Fibrosis of the bladder causes loss of bladder elasticity, which can interfere with urine storage and cause kidney damage.

Abnormal matrix development in young bladders may not be clinically evident until later in life. The cause of this process is largely unexplored.

Men with BPH experience an increase in the connective tissue of the bladder wall in response to the mild obstruction, and men with post-prostatectomy incontinence may have damage to urethral connective tissue. Mature adults often have age-related changes to the bladder and urethral tissue, including increased tissue fragility, decreased elasticity, and alterations in force generation. Neurologically compromised patients may also have bladder dysfunction and associated alterations in connective tissue.

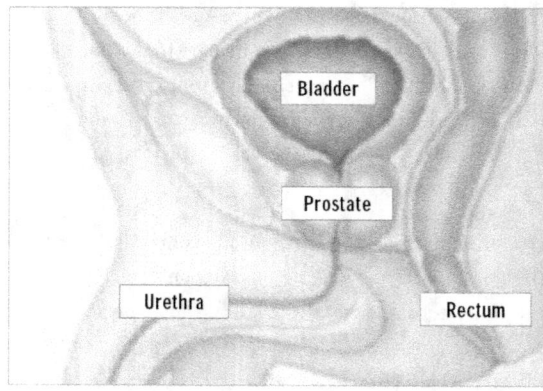

The enlarged prostate gland in benign prostatic hyperplasia or BPH squeezes the urethra, causing an increase in bladder pressure that results in an increase in connective tissue and a subsequent thickening of the bladder wall. (Photo Credit: The American Foundation for Urologic Disease)

Research Advances and Opportunities

A review of the current active portfolio at the National Institutes of Health (NIH) identified a total of 16 grants that partly or fully study connective tissue research; however, none of these grants involves connective tissue of the lower urinary tract. Although several recent advances have been made in the understanding of connective tissue of the lower urinary tract and the role it plays in disorders, much still needs to be done. Immunohistochemistry and gene expression, regeneration, genomics and proteomics, and cell signaling and regulation are discoveries that can be built on to further our understanding of connective tissue function in lower urinary tract disorders.

Immunohistochemistry and Gene Expression

Studies reported in 1996 that bladder dysfunction in pediatric patients is characterized by excessive deposition of several collagen types within the muscle bundles of the bladder wall. Immunohistochemistry has demonstrated that this fibrosis consists of two types of collagen, types I and III. Researchers observed that when collagen gene expression increased, protein deposition increased. This correlation suggests that bladder dysfunction alters gene expression in the cells of the bladder wall. Because they are accompanied by compromised bladder elasticity, these alterations in connective tissue could adversely affect the physiologic function of the bladder.

Regeneration

Another 1996 study suggests that the bladder has an uncanny ability to regenerate. Researchers partially removed the bladders of rats and sutured a tissue matrix devoid of all cellular elements to the defect. The exact composition of this acellular matrix was unknown, but it likely contained collagen, elastin, and other non-cellular matrix elements. Within four days, the epithelium completely covered the acellular matrix, and within two weeks, native smooth muscle was seen streaming into the acellular matrix in association with a new epithelium.

It is hypothesized that cellular interactions between the epithelium, non-cellular matrix, and the embryonic mesenchyme facilitate new growth of smooth muscle.

The ability to use an acellular matrix to regenerate portions of the bladder wall underscores the importance of connective tissue in promoting the normal architectural regeneration of bladder wall tissues and raises the expectation that new therapies will eventually be developed based on this type of research.

Genomics and Proteomics

Research opportunities also exist in the areas of genomics and proteomics. Tissue samples from persons with disorders of the lower urinary tract can be analyzed at the genomics level to characterize global gene expression. Similar types of studies of proteins found in urine and blood and in lower urinary tract tissues can be done in proteomics. Genomics and proteomics may ultimately help to determine

- A common genotype or phenotype that exists for women with stress incontinence

- The genomic and proteomic "fingerprint" of each of the cell types within the lower urinary tract

- Genomic and proteomic fingerprints that can be used to define a "normal" cell phenotype

- Genomic and proteomic fingerprints that differ in males and females, young and old, people with neurogenic bladders, people with Parkinson's disease, and other groups

Cell Regulation and Cell Signaling

The urinary bladder is formed in the embryo from (1) epithelial cells derived from the endoderm and (2) mesenchymal cells derived from the urogenital sinus and allantois. Bladder mesenchyme differentiates into bladder smooth muscle via an unknown signaling mechanism originating from the epithelium. This signaling between the epithelium and mesenchyme hypothetically occurs through diffusion of growth factors.

Supporting this hypothesis is evidence that a number of known growth factors and their receptors are regulated as a function of bladder development and are also modulated during experimental bladder outlet obstruction. Furthermore, growth factors most likely affect degradative proteins in the non-cellular matrix. These proteins play a role in bladder remodeling during development and in partial outlet obstruction. An alternative hypothesis is that signaling in embryonic bladder development occurs via the non-cellular matrix and connective tissue.

Cell signaling also occurs after the bladder has formed, for example during bladder injury. KGF, a growth factor secreted by the bladder's connective tissue framework, is directly responsible for the proliferation of epithelium during bladder injury. KGF acts directly on the epithelium, which harbors the receptor. In humans, bladder epithelium turns over once or twice a year and has the incredible ability to immediately proliferate when injured, covering the exposed areas of bladder muscle and submucosa, the layer of connective tissue underneath the mucous epithelium.

It follows that the ideal cellular lining for the bladder is epithelium. However, for patients requiring bladder enlargement, the bladder is often augmented with intestinal or gastric segments. This procedure creates numerous problems because the tissues that are used are structurally and functionally different from bladder tissue. Studies suggest that cell signaling between the bladder epithelial cells and the intestinal stroma (muscle and non-cellular matrix) leads to changes in the epithelium (urothelium).

This hypothesis was tested by tissue recombination experiments performed by combining rat and mouse rectal mesenchyme and stroma with epithelium from embryonic, newborn, and adult mice or rats, respectively. Both mouse and rat epithelium were changed to a glandular morphology under the influence of rectal mesenchyme. The epithelial transdifferentiation into glandular epithelium was not a function of epithelial age and occurred in the embryonic, newborn, and adult epithelium. Likewise, rectal mesenchyme from embryonic, neonatal, and adult animals induced glandular differentiation in bladder epithelium (urothelium).

In summary, cell signaling is important in bladder development, bladder injury, and bladder regeneration. The components of the bladder—urothelium, extracellular matrix, and muscle, along with nerves and blood vessels—are involved in this signaling process. Elucidating this process is crucial for a better understanding of both normal and abnormal lower urinary tract development.

Specific Opportunities for Connective Tissue Research

Specific opportunities for connective tissue and matrix research exist in the following areas, based on recent research discoveries:

➜ Immunohistochemistry and Gene Expression

- Explore how bladder dysfunction alters gene expression in the cells of the bladder wall

- Determine how alterations in connective tissue adversely affect the physiologic function of the bladder

➜ Regeneration

- Explore how the bladder regenerates

- Determine the cellular interactions among the urothelium, the non-cellular connective tissue matrix, and the mesenchyme that facilitate new growth of smooth muscle

- Develop new therapies involving the use of an acellular matrix to regenerate portions of the bladder wall

➜ Genomics and Proteomics

- Determine whether a common genotype or phenotype exists for persons with stress incontinence

- Identify the genomic and proteomic "fingerprint" of each of the cell types within the lower urinary tract

- Investigate whether genomic and proteomic fingerprints can be used to define a "normal" cell phenotype

- Establish whether genomic and proteomic fingerprints differ in males and females, young and old, people with neurogenic bladders, people with Parkinson's disease, and other groups

➜ Cell Regulation and Cell Signaling

Cell signaling is important in bladder development, bladder injury, and bladder regeneration. The components of the bladder—epithelium, non-cellular connective tissue matrix, muscle, nerves, and blood vessels—are clearly involved in this signaling process. A better understanding of this process is critical to understand both normal and abnormal development.

- Explore cell signaling between the epithelium and mesenchyme that hypothetically occurs through diffusion of growth factors. (According to research evidence, a number of known growth factors and their receptors are regulated as a function of bladder development and are also modulated during experimental bladder outlet obstruction.)

- Investigate the growth factors that most likely affect non-cellular matrix degradative proteins, which play a role in bladder remodeling during development and in partial outlet obstruction

- Explore the alternative hypothesis that signaling in bladder development occurs via the non-cellular matrix and connective tissue

- Determine the role of the non-cellular connective tissue matrix scaffold in the cell signaling that occurs in healing epithelial injury

Future Research Areas

Future research areas important for understanding connective tissue and matrix of the lower urinary tract include cell differentiation and matrix elements, matrix proteins, genomics and proteomics, animal model development, bladder mechanics, gene expression, behavioral techniques, and people with special needs.

Cell Differentiation and Matrix Elements

Future research on the lower urinary tract must define the elements that maintain the differentiative state of cell types within the lower urinary tract and pelvic floor. Tissue engineers and other researchers who study the effects of obstruction, aging, and pathology on the bladder would benefit from information about matrix elements. Questions for researchers are as follows:

- What factors control the phenotypic stability of individual cell types in the bladder, urinary sphincter, ureter, and pelvic floor?

- Are these factors age-, hormone-, cytokine-, or sex-dependent?

- What is the role of the non-cellular connective tissue matrix in maintaining cellular phenotype? Does the matrix change with age?

- Does the matrix sequester cytokines, hormones, and other factors that influence cellular type?

- What signals emanating from the matrix influence the epithelium?

- Do integrins—non-cellular matrix receptors that play a role in cell adhesion—alter cell behavior? If so, which integrins, and do these types of interactions change with pathology, with aging, and during development?

- What is the role of the epithelial and smooth muscle basement membranes in maintaining cellular phenotype?

- How do cells interact with the matrix?

- Are there specific receptors for domains within individual matrix macromolecules?

- How are such receptors acquired? Do they become altered in disease?

- What are the basic elements of cell-matrix interactions?

- How does the matrix control smooth muscle cell differentiation? What molecules are involved?

- Can these events be duplicated using stem cells or other forms of undifferentiated cells?

Matrix Proteins

Little is know about the function of protein fragments derived from matrix proteins. These types of fragments can be generated by a variety of mechanisms that decompose proteins and might be expected to have profound biological activities. Questions for research to answer are as follows:

- Does degradation of the matrix lead to phenotypic modulation of cells that interact with degraded matrix components?

- What types of materials involved in degradation are normally present within the normal bladder, the developing bladder, and the diseased bladder?

- How are these enzymes modulated?

- Does age alter the normal complement of degradative enzymes present?

- Does the hormonal environment alter these same degradative enzymes?

- What types of matrix macromolecules do all cell types in the bladder produce?

Genomics and Proteomics

Genomic and proteomic studies of tissue-specific gene and protein expression would provide valuable information on the specific complement of genes and proteins that defines bladder, urethral, ureteral, and pelvic floor tissues.

Animal Model Development

Another potentially valuable area is the development of animal models to study interactions between the mesenchyme and the epithelium. Questions that research needs to answer are as follows:

- Are certain types of chemical compounds sequestered within the matrix?

- What are the causes of urinary incontinence and pelvic organ prolapse in women?

- What behavioral therapies (e.g., stretching and strengthening exercises) will help women maintain normal connective tissue?

- Does diet, including vitamin C, improve post-operative outcome and overall connective tissue strength?

Bladder Mechanics

Little is known about the manner in which the bladder can mechanically accommodate large-volume variations. Questions for research include:

- How are the mucosal and bladder muscle (detrusor) layers connected?

- Can these connections be mechanically characterized?

- What is the three-dimensional structure of the bladder wall in both health and disease?

- How is tension generated through the interactions of the proteins, actin and myosin conveyed across the cell membrane to the non-cellular matrix and to other tissue layers in the bladder wall?

Gene Expression

The ability to evaluate gene expression at the cell-type, tissue, and organ level is also lacking in lower urinary tract research. Some of the problems in this area are technology-based and concern the inability or difficulty individual researchers have in accessing appropriate technology to carry out high throughput (the number of tests that can be performed in a given period of time) experiments at the cellular and molecular levels. For example, tissue-specific and cell-type-specific marker proteins for lower urinary tract cells are largely unknown. With the appropriate characterization of individual cell types within the bladder wall, pelvic floor, and other structures of the lower urinary tract, characterization can be accomplished. This characterization will lead to the development of specific reagents and cDNA probes to permit further refinement of the traits of each of the cell types unique to the structures and tissues being studied.

The development of these tools will enhance the research capabilities of investigators and permit them to use genomic and proteomic tools to formulate hypothesis–driven research. Such tools are being made available to researchers of other organ systems, and similar efforts should be undertaken to ensure that bladder research successfully takes advantage of information provided by the Human Genome Project.

Behavioral Techniques

Questions for future behavioral research are as follows:

- Can behavioral techniques such as biofeedback and exercise improve urinary function?

- Are there behavioral manifestations of the aging process that affect urination?

- Does exercise improve the long-term health and physiologic function of the lower urinary tract?

People with Special Needs

Connective tissue research directed at groups of patients with special needs is also important. These groups include

- Children with lower urinary tract disorders that may predispose them to kidney damage

- Adults with spinal cord injury or other illnesses that compromise lower urinary tract function

- Aging adults who show progressive deterioration of urinary function and its associated morbidity

- People with diabetes

- Women with interstitial cystitis

- Women at risk for developing urinary incontinence and pelvic organ prolapse

In regard to the latter, research on rectal prolapse has indicated that joint mobility might be a possible marker for connective tissue abnormalities of the lower urinary tract.

In addition, there is a great need to understand the molecular changes that occur in the connective tissue of pregnant women. Connective tissue of the uterus increases tenfold during pregnancy, then disappears within a few weeks after childbirth. With pregnancy, women often experience the simultaneous onset of urinary tract infections. Because joint mobility is well documented during pregnancy and resolves after childbirth, some bladder injury involving damage to connective tissue might occur during childbirth.

Investigations into using the presence of striae, bands of connective tissue that appear on the abdomen of some pregnant women, and joint mobility as indicators or markers of potential connective tissue damage might reveal information that would motivate clinicians to modify the mode of delivery and prevent bladder injury during childbirth.

CHAPTER 3

MUSCLE

Basic Science of the Lower Urinary Tract

DID YOU KNOW?

→ Many diseases and conditions such as diabetes, Parkinson's disease, stroke, and multiple sclerosis have a significant impact on bladder muscle.

→ Failure of bladder muscle to function properly can lead to recurrent infection, incontinence, urine retention, voiding dysfunction, irreversible muscle failure, and disease in other parts of the urinary tract such as the kidney.

Summary and Recommendations

Understanding normal muscle structure and function and the changes that lead to bladder disease is critically important to public health. However, compared with the current understanding of other muscle types, such as those of the heart or blood vessels, the understanding of lower urinary tract muscle is woefully inadequate. Poor funding and lack of research in this area have contributed substantially to this situation.

To improve prevention and treatment of lower urinary tract disorders, more research must be done to elucidate the functions of normal myocytes—the cells that form muscle—and to understand the impact of age and disease on these cells. Correction of altered muscle cell function can correct the symptoms of bladder dysfunction; therefore, the Bladder Research Progress Review Group recommends that the National Institutes of Health (NIH)

→ **Conduct more basic studies of the muscle structure and function of the urinary and reproductive systems, including studies of**

- Biomechanics

- Comparative muscle physiology (i.e., urethral smooth muscle versus bladder smooth muscle; urethral sphincter versus rectal sphincter)

- Characteristics of receptor and effector pharmacology and cell signal transduction in smooth muscle of the urinary and reproductive tracts

- Three-dimensional anatomy and its correlation with function

➡ Conduct more molecular, cellular, and tissue investigations into lower urinary tract muscle deterioration and failure. Examples of interesting modulatory factors to be studied include

- Nerve factors

- Growth factors

- Programmed cell death (apoptosis)

- Progenitor cells (i.e., stem cells)

- Trauma (i.e., vaginal delivery)

- Hormones

- Aging

- Development

➡ Develop new imaging technologies and apply non-invasive methods from other fields (e.g., cardiology) to assess muscle function in the body

➡ Conduct studies of the basic disease mechanisms, prevention, and treatment of end-stage bladder failure

➡ Investigate smooth and skeletal muscle stem cells, their role in normal development, and their use in regeneration

Background

Because the bladder is predominantly a muscular organ, muscle disorders are common and clinically significant. Failure of the bladder muscle to function properly can lead to infection, incontinence, urine retention, voiding dysfunction, irreversible muscle failure, and disease in other parts of the urinary tract such as the kidney.

Muscle tissue, like other tissue, is composed of cells and non-cellular substance located outside the cells. Muscle cells or myocytes are elongated and are called fibers. These fibers are embedded in areolar connective tissue.

Normal Bladder Muscle

The normal, unstretched bladder has muscle bundles or fascicles of varying sizes, lengths, and orientation that are surrounded by a collagen sheet. Connecting the fascicles to each other are wavy collagen bundles that form helical coils, which lengthen and thin during distention of the intact bladder. Running as geodesic lines around the bladder, the muscle fascicles cover the shortest distance between two points, sometimes leaving discontinuities.

Elastin has also been found on the surface of muscle fascicles. Bundled and surrounded by collagen and elastin layers, the muscle fascicles can move independently, which allows them to contract freely. In addition, this bundled structure allows for large stretches to occur in the bladder wall.

Bladder muscle has three layers: an inner longitudinal layer, a middle circular layer, and an outer longitudinal layer. Where the bladder opens into the urethra, the circular fibers are thick and form a sphincter muscle that is normally in a state of contraction. The sphincter relaxes only when nerves, reacting to the accumulation of a quantity of urine, send signals to the brain that it is necessary to release the urine. Disorders affecting the muscle of the bladder wall often affect the ureters and the bladder outlet, and vice versa.

Bladder muscle, like all muscle, has several distinguishing characteristics:

- Irritability (excitability)—muscle cells receive stimuli and, like all cells, respond to it

- Contractility—muscle cells can change shape and become shorter

- Extensibility—muscle cells can stretch

- Elasticity—muscle cells can readily return to their original form when the stretching force is removed

Because the underlying epithelium, nerves, and blood-borne hormones and modulators, including urine substances under certain conditions, can affect bladder muscle cells, diverse arrays of cell signaling mechanisms can affect the physiology of the muscle cell as well. In addition, more than one receptor-effector system is likely to be activated at any point in time in any given muscle cell.

Research on smooth muscle has indicated that regional hormonal mechanisms may be involved in the stretch-evoked release of excitatory substances from smooth muscle and that these substances may drive smooth muscle activity. This type of research could have a major impact on conditions that involve instability of the bladder muscle, which can cause incontinence.

Muscle Dysfunction

The bladder is predominantly a muscular organ. Disorders of the bladder and urethral sphincter are common and of significant clinical importance. Bladder muscle dysfunction can lead to infection, incontinence, urine retention, voiding dysfunction, and eventually, irreversible muscle failure or end-stage bladder failure. Other parts of the urinary tract such as the kidney may also eventually be affected.

Common symptoms of bladder muscle dysfunction and other lower urinary tract muscle disorders are

- Frequency and urgency

- Incontinence and pelvic floor disorders

- Urine retention (i.e., end-stage bladder failure)

- Upper urinary tract diseases, such as hydronephrosis (blockage)

- Bladder muscle overactivity

In turn, aging and various disease states affect the detrusor muscle of the bladder and its associated lower urinary tract musculature. Some primary diseases and conditions are

- Diabetes mellitus

- Injury from therapies such as radiation and surgery

- Neurologic dysfunction (hypocontractility) resulting from multiple sclerosis, Parkinsonism spinal cord injury, stroke, and developmental anomalies

- Overactive bladder (hypercontractility), detrusor muscle instability (with or without impaired contractility), and pelvic floor disorders

- Interstitial cystitis

- Obstruction caused by benign enlargement of the prostate gland (benign prostatic hyperplasia or BPH) and prostate cancer

- Effects of vaginal delivery

- Vascular injury

Research Advances and Opportunities

Advances

Studies have been underway to develop gene therapy for stress incontinence. The concept behind this potential therapy is to build up the deficient urethral sphincter muscle. To achieve this, tissue engineering or cell-based *ex vivo* gene therapy appears to be more logical than conventional viral vector gene therapy. According to one study, muscle-derived, cell-based tissue engineering (autologous cell transplantation) may have several advantages over the current treatment for urinary incontinence—bovine collagen injection.

The advantage of autologous cell transplantation is that the transplanted cells will not cause an immune system or allergic reaction and, therefore, will survive longer than injected collagen, which is derived from cows. Transplanted cells can also serve as a natural bulking agent when injected into the bladder and urethra, and they may form muscle fibers that become part of the host muscle. Therefore, the transplanted cells serve as a blocking agent and are physiologically capable of improving bladder (detrusor) muscle contractility.

A study of this technique demonstrated three facts in the emerging field of urologic tissue engineering:

- Injecting skeletal-muscle-derived cells into the urethal sphincter is feasible

- Gene transfer to the bladder and urethra is feasible

- Injected human-muscle-derived collagen has greater persistence than injected bovine collagen

In the autologous cell transplantation procedure currently being developed to construct functionally and anatomically normal, tissue-engineered bladders, bladder urothelial and muscle cells newly isolated from an animal attached to biodegradable matrices (scaffolds) *in vitro*. When implanted *in vivo*, these cells reorganized into multi-layered structures. After implantation, the supporting cell matrix became vascularized in concert with expansion of the cell mass, thereby allowing cell survival by diffusion of nutrients across short distances.

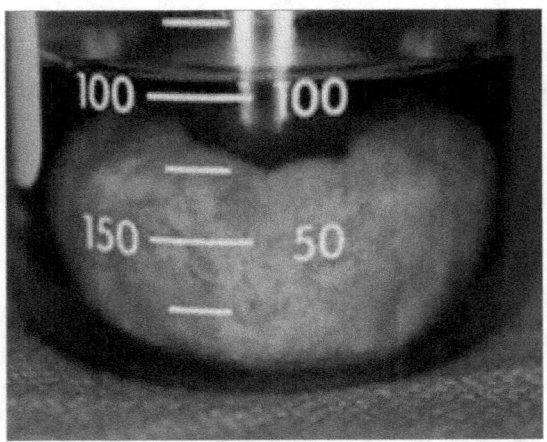

A bladder engineered in the laboratory. *(Photo Credit: Dr. Anthony Atala, Children's Hospital and Harvard Medical School.)*

Gene therapy has also recently achieved several important milestones with the development of tissue engineered for bladder replacement using a small intestine scaffold seeded with bladder smooth muscle and epithelium. In another development, cartilage cells were injected for the treatment of stress incontinence and vesicoureteral reflux. Urge incontinence is another disorder that would benefit from gene therapy.

Possible gene therapy strategies for overactive bladders and urge incontinence may include suppression of bladder muscle activity or neural pathways that trigger the micturition (voiding) reflex.

Opportunities

Research on lower urinary tract muscles has provided numerous opportunities for furthering our understanding of lower urinary tract diseases. Research opportunities exist in

- Neuromodulation treatment of hyperactive and underactive bladder muscle disorders.

- Magnetic resonance imaging (MRI) for detection of abnormalities in levator muscles.

- Data on the fine structure underlying overactivity and underactivity of bladder muscle in older adults.

- Improved understanding of smooth (visceral) and striated (skeletal) muscle physiology and cell biology in other organs; this understanding could be applied to the lower urinary tract in the future.

- Evidence that the striated muscle within the urethra deteriorates at twice the rate present in other striated muscles and is accompanied by the loss of intramuscular nerve axons. Also, a great many variations exist in the number of viable fibers present among persons of the same age.

Understanding normal muscle structure, function, and the changes that lead to bladder disease is of critical importance to public health. Unfortunately, compared with the current understanding of other muscle types such as those of the heart or blood vessels, the understanding of lower urinary tract muscle is woefully inadequate. To improve prevention and treatment of lower urinary tract disorders, more research must be done to elucidate the functions of normal muscle cells and to understand the impact of age and disease on these cells.

CHAPTER 4

NERVES AND BLOOD VESSELS

Basic Science of the Lower Urinary Tract

DID YOU KNOW?

→ Diseases and conditions of the nervous system such as spinal cord injury, multiple sclerosis, and Parkinson's are highly associated with lower urinary tract dysfunction.

→ The specific or separate role of nerves and blood vessels in the development of lower urinary tract disorders is currently deficient or unknown and requires significantly more research.

→ Possible gene therapy strategies for overactive bladders and urge incontinence may include suppression of nerve pathways that trigger the micturition (voiding or urination) reflex.

→ Preliminary studies have also been done to determine the benefits of gene therapy for overflow incontinence caused by diabetic neurogenic bladder dysfunction and interstitial cystitis (IC) and for bladder pain caused by IC.

Summary and Recommendations

Research on how the nervous system and vascular system influence dysfunctions of the lower urinary tract has many potentially important avenues for progress. In the past decade, a major emphasis on research in neuroscience has advanced (1) knowledge about peripheral nerves and their relationship with peripheral organs and (2) knowledge about the central nervous system (CNS) and how it changes. These advances may have specific applications for research projects that study the lower urinary tract.

The development of transgenic models may also be necessary. Transgenic models are organisms in which new DNA has been introduced into the germ cells by injection into the nucleus of the ovum (gene transplant). Some transgenic animal models already available for different disease states are of relevance to the bladder. These models could be used to determine whether it is possible to minimize the effect of injury to nerves or to accelerate their healing with such things as hormonal substances and nerve growth factors.

Based on a review of the current research portfolio at the National Institutes of Health (NIH), the Bladder Research Progress Review Group has made the following specific high priority recommendations for increased research funding and resources:

➡ Improve assessment and quantification of neural function of the lower urinary tract.

➡ Improve knowledge of nerve cell-target interactions, endothelial factors, and epithelial factors

➡ Improve basic anatomic and physiologic information on gender and aging differences in neural pathways involved in voiding (micturition)

➡ Develop strategies to protect nerves during critical life events and investigate neurotrophic factors and nerve regeneration in the lower urinary tract

➡ Improve basic anatomic and physiologic information concerning the impact of blood supply on lower urinary tract function

- → Advance genomics and proteomics technologies

- → Develop novel therapies, technologies, and gene therapy for lower urinary tract disorders

- → Define the neurotransmission principles unique to lower urinary tract function

Background

Normal functioning of the lower urinary tract depends on intact and appropriate coordination of nerves in the central and peripheral nervous systems. Unlike other organ systems, the lower urinary tract absolutely requires this coordinated control. The lower urinary tract must also receive a blood supply that is not only adequate, but also highly regulated and modulated.

As a result, the lower urinary tract is affected by a wide spectrum of circumstances and life events, many of which have a basis in the nervous and vascular systems, that interact and are interdependent in the lower urinary tract. Pertinent examples include, but are not limited to, degenerative diseases of the nervous system such as Alzheimer's and Parkinson's, spinal cord injury, maternal birth trauma, diabetes, multiple sclerosis, benign prostatic hyperplasia (BPH), post-surgical events in both males and females, pelvic radiation therapy, and urinary incontinence. Spinal cord injury, multiple sclerosis, and Parkinson's disease in particular are highly associated with lower urinary tract dysfunction. The specific or separate role of vascular factors in the development of lower urinary tract disorders is currently unknown and requires significantly more research.

Because they play a central role in lower urinary tract function, the nervous and vascular systems are also involved in virtually every disorder or problem of the lower urinary tract. If these problems are to be overcome and even prevented, the neurovascular influences must be vigorously investigated.

Development of Bladder Control

The neurophysiologic mechanism of normal bladder control involves bladder storage of urine and voluntary evacuation. This mechanism is controlled by a complex integration of sympathetic, parasympathetic, and somatic innervation that involves the lower urinary tract, the sacral spinal cord, the midbrain, and higher cortical centers of the brain.

Voiding starts in the fetus and is mainly by reflex at frequent intervals. Bladder filling triggers afferent (inflowing) nerves that, through spinal reflexes, cause relaxation of the external urinary sphincter. This results in complete emptying of the bladder. By the time a child is six months of age, bladder capacity has increased and the frequency of voiding has decreased.

Between one and two years of age, conscious sensation develops, and by two to three years of age, the ability to initiate and inhibit voiding from the cerebral cortex develops. At this time the lower urinary tract is most susceptible to abnormal, learned input into the cerebral cortex. This input may be as simple as telling a child not to wet his or her pants, no matter what—a command that may lead to either appropriate socialization or a pathologic failure to relax the sphincter when it is appropriate.

Storage and periodic voiding of urine by the bladder requires coordinated and appropriate input from the nervous system. The elements of the nervous system involved in lower urinary tract control include

- Peripheral nerves in the bladder and in the wall of the urethra

- Autonomic (organ) and voluntary (skeletal) sensory and motor nerves and ganglia

- Local (segmental) spinal circuits

- Long-loop connections to the brain stem (pons) micturition center, the center that controls urination

- Reciprocal connections between the cerebral cortex, the brain autonomic centers (centers that regulate nerve impulses activating smooth muscles of organs and glands), and the brain stem micturition center

Unfortunately, the current state of knowledge about neurovascular influences is extremely deficient. Current behavioral, pharmacologic, and surgical treatments of lower urinary tract disorders arising from problems in the nervous system are often inadequate, cause complications, and fail to eradicate the underlying condition.

In addition, drugs used to manage these disorders are restricted to compounds that affect neurotransmission only in the peripheral nervous system (e.g., anticholinergics and alpha-adrenergic antagonists). More effective and innovative approaches are needed.

Nervous system and vascular system contributions to disorders of the lower urinary tract may be amenable to prevention or early intervention efforts. Certain conditions such as spinal cord injury are receiving intense research funding, and collaboration with researchers in these areas may elucidate information that will enhance optimal lower urinary tract function in afflicted individuals. For example, well-studied progressive diseases of the nervous or vascular systems may provide an opportunity to develop prevention or early intervention programs that could reduce lower urinary tract malfunction. Also, identifying modifiable obstetric practices may reduce maternal birth injury, a cause of urinary incontinence. These are high-yield areas for research funding with immediate opportunities for translational research and rapid clinical impact.

Research Advances and Opportunities

In the past decade, a major emphasis on research in neuroscience has advanced knowledge about the peripheral nervous system and the organs it serves and about the central nervous system (CNS) and how it changes. These advances may have specific applications for research projects that study the lower urinary tract. Several important avenues for progress have developed recently, including studies on brain imaging, biochemistry of the nervous system, interactions between nerve cells and target organs, nerve protection and preservation, nerve regeneration, neurotrophic factors, blood supply, genomics and proteomics technologies, gene therapy and tissue engineering, and development of transgenic models.

Brain Imaging

Recently, interest has focused on using new brain imaging methods to obtain insight into normal voiding, to localize brain abnormalities associated with incontinence, or to determine the site of action of pharmaceutical agents.

These new methods rely on changes in the metabolism or oxygen use of nerve cells in the brain to assess their function during urination. When active, the nerve cells use more oxygen and activate metabolic pathways whose constituents can be monitored. When a person voids or attempts to hold urine, very specific sites within the brain and spinal cord are activated. These areas behave differently as a person ages or if the brain has been injured from lack of oxygen caused by obstruction of its blood supply.

Studies in humans indicate that voluntary control of voiding is dependent on (1) connections between the frontal cortex of the cerebrum and a region of the hypothalamus and (2) connections between a small lobe near the center of the cerebral cortex (the paracentral lobule) and the brain stem. Lesions in these areas of the cerebral cortex appear to increase bladder activity directly by removing the cortex's inhibitory control. Brain imaging studies in human volunteers have implicated two areas of the cerebrum—the frontal cortex and the anterior cingulate gyrus—as the areas of the brain that control urination and have indicated that urination is controlled predominantly by the right side of the brain. Gyri are the prominent, rounded elevations that form the cerebral hemispheres.

Positron emission tomography (PET) has been used on human subjects to determine which brain areas are involved in human micturition (urination). According to one study,

- Urination was associated with increased blood flow in four areas of the brain (the right dorsomedial pontine tegmentum, the periaqueductal grey, the hypothalamus, and the right inferior frontal gyrus)

- Withholding urine was associated with decreased blood flow in the right anterior cingulate gyrus of the cerebrum

- Unsuccessful attempts to urinate were associated with increased blood flow in the right ventral pontine tegmentum of the brain stem, an area that according to animal studies appears to control the motor neurons innervating the pelvic floor, and in the right inferior frontal gyrus of the cerebrum.

These results suggest that the human brain stem contains specific nuclei responsible for the control of urination, and that the regions for micturition in the brain stem and the cerebral cortex are predominantly on the right side of the brain.

The results of the PET study were in accordance with the results of a clinical study of patients with chronic paralysis of one side of the body (hemiplegia). In this study, which dealt with the chronic sequelae of stroke, frequency and urgency of urination occurred more commonly in patients with lesions of the right hemisphere. Such studies are extremely useful in delineating normal and abnormal processes in the brain that are associated with bladder disorders. With further study, these techniques may be useful for diagnosis or for planning therapy.

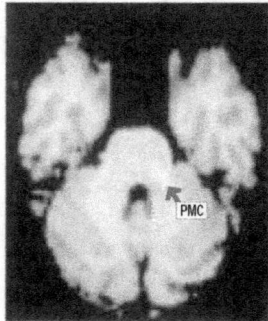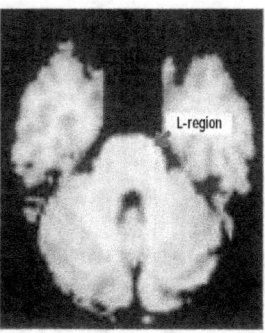

Increased activation of areas in the brain on positron emission tomography (PET scan), **left**, with voiding, **right**, with attempts to hold urine. (*Photo Credit: Dr. Bertil Blok, University of Groningen, Groningen, Netherlands*)

Another PET study, conducted in adult female volunteers, identified brain structures involved in the voluntary motor control of the pelvic floor during rest, repetitive pelvic floor straining, sustained pelvic floor straining, and sustained abdominal straining. The results revealed that two sections of the cerebrum are activated during contraction of the abdominal muscles: the superomedial precentral gyrus (the most medial portion of the cerebrum's motor cortex) and the superolateral precentral gyrus, also in the cerebrum. Significant activations were found in the cerebellum, the supplementary motor cortex, and the thalamus as well. The portion of the cerebrum known as the right anterior cingulate gyrus was activated during sustained pelvic floor straining.

Normal urethral sphincter function appears to be present in stroke victims whose lesions are restricted to the basal ganglia or thalamus. When these patients sensed an impending involuntary bladder contraction or its onset, they were able to voluntarily contract the sphincter muscle and stop, or considerably lessen, the effect of the abnormal urination reflex. Under the same circumstances, people with lesions in the cerebral cortex or internal capsule, the layer of white matter that connects the cortex to the brain stem, were unable to forcefully contract the sphincter muscle. Thus, they have a profound abnormality in the cerebral-to-corticospinal circuitry necessary for voluntary control of the sphincter muscle.

Biochemistry Studies

A variety of autonomic system disorders and emotional disorders such as depression and anxiety are associated with changes within the prefrontal cortex, the area of the cerebrum responsible for biologic intelligence. Because many emotional states are associated with overactive bladder, neurochemical changes within this area of the brain may also have an impact on a range of voiding dysfunctions.

Studies of the biochemical process that activates serotonin, a neurotransmitter that stimulates bladder smooth muscle, have determined that the serotonin-activating system plays a major role in voiding as well as in emotional states such as depression, anxiety, and eating disorders. Differences between men and women in the operation of the serotonin-activating system may explain why certain psychiatric disorders such as depression, anorexia, and bulimia, and certain disorders of the lower urinary tract are more common in women.

Women have substantially lower levels of 5-HT than men do. This substance is involved in the production of serotonin. In one study using PET scans, areas of the brain that demonstrated lowered 5-HT function corresponded to areas of the brain that had a decreased blood supply when subjects were instructed to hold urine. Data from several studies circumstantially support a role for reduced 5-HT activity or receptor function, hormonal influences, and linkage between brain sites for depression, hyperactive voiding, and altered 5-HT activity. Studies such as these may help direct and monitor drug development for bladder disorders.

Interactions between Nerve Cells and Target Organs

Recent studies have revealed that communication between nerves and their target organs is not unidirectional, as previously thought. The nervous system and target organs have a chemical dialogue that is essential for the normal functioning of the lower urinary tract, as well as for adaptation to pathological conditions. This dialogue, if dysfunctional, could contribute to a variety of urinary tract disorders.

Various examples of non-traditional, nerve-target organ interactions in the urinary bladder have been identified, including

* Alterations in afferent nerves and efferent nerves caused by neurotrophic factors (factors involved in the nutrition and metabolism of nerve cells) that are released from smooth muscle cells in the enlarged and thickened bladder wall.

* Chemical communication between cells of the bladder's epithelium and afferent nerves

* Chemical interactions between afferent nerves and mast cells during inflammation

A more detailed understanding of the mechanisms underlying two-way neuron-target organ communication would provide new insights into the pathophysiologic mechanisms underlying voiding dysfunction and identify new molecules and pathways as targets for drug therapy.

Nerve Protection, Preservation, and Regeneration Studies

Research on nerve protection, preservation, and regeneration has advanced rapidly in recent years and is the outcome of allocation of research resources to these areas, based on the needs of patients affected by stroke, neurodegenerative diseases, nervous system trauma, and pediatric developmental abnormalities, and also on the recognition that the nervous system is particularly susceptible to the damaging effects of the ischemia-reperfusion cycle. In this cycle, tissue is injured because obstructed blood flow reduces the supply of oxygen to the cells (ischemia) and further damage occurs when the blood supply is restored (reperfusion injury).

Very little of this information has been applied directly to research affecting the lower urinary tract. A notable exception is the currently supported effort to deliver neurotrophic genes (i.e., nerve growth factor or NGF) to the lower urinary tract to treat the effects of diabetes. NGF has been found to play a significant role in the support, maintenance, and phenotype of many bladder peripheral efferent nerves. NGF also prevents programmed cell death (apoptosis) of nerve cells stressed by obstructed blood flow (ischemia) and reperfusion events as well as by nerve toxins.

Neurotrophic Factors

Knowledge about the relationship between neurotrophic factor action and apoptotic cell death in the nervous system has advanced rapidly in the past few years. Specific strategies have been developed to ameliorate and prevent the induction of programmed nerve cell death caused by a variety of stresses and events. Very little is known regarding the impact of specific life events on nerve cell death and function in the lower urinary tract or how this may be altered.

Blood Supply

Normal bladder function depends on the delivery of an adequate supply of blood and nutrients to the bladder mucous tissue, muscle, and nerves. Recent research evidence indicates that several dysfunctions of the urinary and reproductive tracts are linked to reduced blood flow and the subsequent decreased oxygen supply to the cells. Examples include diabetic bladder disorder, obstructive bladder disease, and bladder muscle instability and loss of elasticity.

Genomics and Proteomics Technologies

A goal of the Human Genome Project is the cataloging of all human cDNA sequences. One result of this effort has been the evolution of functional genomics, a science that will deepen the biologic understanding of human physiology and disease through the total elucidation of gene function in both normal and pathophysiologic states.

The DNA microarray is the first effective, rapid, and nearly universally applicable tool of functional genomics to be used for unraveling mechanisms of cell function and disease pathogenesis at the whole-genome scale. The advent of DNA microarray technology has been heralded as the beginning of a new epoch in biomedical research principally because this technology is easily integrated both operationally and conceptually into ongoing research projects.

These evolving technologies hold the promise to provide insights ranging from predispositions to lower urinary tract dysfunctions, to the targeting of specific therapies to responsive patient subgroups, to the idiosyncratic handling of drugs. Such data may provide markers (a characteristic or factor by which a cell or molecule can be recognized or identified) for use in early detection and prevention strategies or gene promoters, which would allow selective targeting to the lower urinary tract.

Gene Therapy and Tissue Engineering

Possible gene therapy strategies for overactive bladders and urge incontinence may include suppression of bladder muscle activity or neural pathways that trigger the micturition (voiding) reflex. It is also plausible that gene transfer of inhibitory neurotransmitters into the bladder and bladder afferent pathways can suppress the urination reflex, thereby inhibiting bladder hyperactivity. In addition, because NGF has been implicated as a chemical mediator to induce overactive bladders in various pathological conditions, such as spinal cord injury, urethral obstruction, and chronic bladder inflammation, antibody-based gene therapy to suppress NGF expression is a potential therapy for the treatment of urge incontinence.

Preliminary studies have also been done to determine the benefits of gene therapy for overflow incontinence caused by diabetic neurogenic bladder dysfunction and interstitial cystitis (IC) and for bladder pain caused by IC.

Transgenic Models

Some transgenic animal models, animals in which new DNA has been introduced into germ cells by injection into the nucleus of the ovum (gene transplant), are already available for different disease states of relevance to the bladder. These models could be used in future studies to determine whether it is possible to minimize the effect of injury to nerves or to accelerate their healing with such things as hormonal substances and nerve growth factors.

Future Research

Assessment and Quantification of Nerve Function

Despite the preeminent role of nerves in urination and in maintaining continence, assessing whether nerves are functioning properly relies on indirect measurements. Electrodiagnostic tests such as electromyography (EMG) offer little more than a detailed physical examination. An EMG is difficult to perform, lacks sensitivity, and is costly. More sensitive and accurate tests are needed to ascertain whether difficulties in voiding or in urine loss arise from abnormalities in muscles versus nerves. Questions that need to be answered in this area are as follows:

- What issues, such as chronic pain and trauma, are specific to the bladder and what clinical situations need to be addressed?

- Why do some patients, even without a neuropathologic process or diabetes, lose the ability to contract the bladder? How can this be prevented or treated more effectively?

- How can we determine whether a problem is caused by afferent (inflowing) fibers, efferent (outflowing) fibers, or the nerve?

- Based on imaging, what are the pain pathways outside the bladder? What are the pain pathways inside the bladder?

- Can imaging be used to explore serotonin transporters and other genes?

- Can specific drugs be used to investigate specific nerve and neuromuscular pathways?

- Are specific drugs for receptor subtypes useful in investigating the role of these receptors in bladder and urethral function?

- What techniques should be used in clinical trials to measure neural milieu in patients?

- What imaging technique should be used to clinically characterize patients?

- How are we to understand or address issues of nervous system control? How can these issues be studied in humans?

- How can neuroscientists be attracted to study the lower urinary tract?

- What are appropriate models for nerve research?

- Is the rat bladder model used in a number of experiments applicable to humans?

Neuron-Target-Organ Interactions, Endothelial and Epithelial Factors

A more detailed understanding of the mechanisms underlying two-way neuron-target organ communication is needed to answer the following questions:

- What are the disease-causing physiological mechanisms underlying voiding dysfunction?

- Are there new molecules and pathways that can be used as targets for drug therapy?

Gender and Aging Differences in Micturition Pathways

In the next few decades, dollars spent in management of these bladder problems will significantly increase for two reasons:

- The proportion of the aged population in the United States is increasing each year with the maturation of the so-called "baby-boomers."

- The prevalence of voiding dysfunction such as urinary incontinence and overactive bladder increases significantly with age.

Unfortunately, most of the financial resources for bladder problems are relegated to hygienic protection (diapers and pads) and not to research and medical treatment of this pressing problem. Our understanding of the basic changes in nerve pathways related to aging

is embarrassingly inadequate to make significant improvement in the voiding dysfunction of the aged population at this juncture in time.

In addition, before age 65, urinary incontinence and overactive bladder are significantly more prevalent in females compared with males. It is not well understood why this is so and whether it is from childbirth or hormonal (estrogen) status. Estrogen can modulate nerve circuitry; therefore, this hormone possibly affects the nerve pathways regulating urination and continence.

It follows that one of the priorities for neurovascular research of the lower urinary tract must be to improve our understanding of the effect of aging and gender on nerves as well as on blood vessels in the lower urinary tract. By understanding these mechanisms, we can increase the quality of life and also the efficiency of health care dollars spent.

Answers to the following critical questions will advance our understanding in this area:

- How many motor nerve nuclei are in the bladder of an adult woman? Of an adult man? Do these nuclei decrease with time?

- Why are women affected disproportionately by bladder disorders? Is it because of the structure of the lower urinary tract in women? Is it hormonal? Is it because of life events such as childbirth? Are there gender-specific aspects of bladder nerve circuits?

- What are the genetics of nerve degeneration in the elderly?

- What happens to bladder nerves with aging?

- How do degenerative diseases of the nervous system have an impact on bladder function?

- Can preventative measures (medical, pharmacological, and physical) prevent voiding changes that occur with aging?

- How does sensory perception of bladder fullness change with age? Is it a function of gender?

Funding research issues related to these areas will increase not only our knowledge, but also the quality of life of many people. Health care expenditures will decrease as a result.

Neurotrophic Factors and Nerve Regeneration

Our understanding of the relationship between the neurotrophic factors, action, and apoptotic cell death in the nervous system has witnessed rapid recent advances. This advancement includes the development of specific strategies to ameliorate and prevent the induction of apoptosis in nerves that is caused by a variety of stresses and events. Very little is known regarding the impact of specific life events on nerve cell death and function in the lower urinary tract or how this may be altered. Questions that research should endeavor to answer are as follows:

- What specific damage to the control of nerves in the lower urinary tract might be prevented by nerve-protective intervention and in what situations? Based on what animal models?

- What other neurotrophic factors are important in the lower urinary tract?

- Is it possible to capitalize on biological mechanisms governing nerve growth and regeneration to ameliorate or reverse damage to the nerve circuits of the lower urinary tract?

- Do some persons lack mechanisms that support post-traumatic or post-surgical nerve recovery? Does nerve-supportive therapy improve outcomes?

Impact of Blood Supply

Recent research evidence indicates that several dysfunctions of the urinary and reproductive tracts are linked to obstructed blood flow and the resulting decreased oxygen supply to the cells (ischemia). Urogenital dysfunctions responsible for this include diabetic bladder disease, obstructive bladder disease, and instability and loss of elasticity in bladder muscle (detrusor). Questions that need to be answered are as follows:

- What is the pathophysiology of ischemia-induced nervous system disorders of the bladder?

- Is there hard evidence to show that reduced oxygen or some element of ischemia actually leads to nerve damage?

- What is the relation between degree and duration of ischemia and neuropathy?

- How does the bladder vasculature adapt to repeated distension and contraction?

- Are there differences between bladders of men and women with respect to the susceptibility to ischemia?

- What is the effect of high pressure in, and over-distension of, the bladder on blood flow and nerve integrity?

- How does ischemic reperfusion cause bladder structural damage and dysfunction?

- Does aging correlate with differential susceptibility to atherosclerotic change?

- What is the anatomy and physiology of blood supply in the human bladder?

- How is blood flow to the bladder regulated?

- What is the role of anoxia (absence of oxygen in blood and tissues) in inducing bladder wall damage?

- Does atherosclerosis affect certain vascular beds more than others?

- Are there risk factors that contribute to bladder ischemia such as smoking, hypertension, and diabetes?

- Is blood flow altered during aging or as a result of other diseases?

- Are there racial differences in susceptibility to ischemia?

- Can nerve regulation of blood flow affect disorders?

- What is the role of nitric oxide in the regulation of blood flow under normal and pathological conditions?

- Can pharmacological alteration of peripheral blood flow be effective in the treatment of specific bladder pathologies?

- What is the effect of radiation on genitourinary blood flow?

- What is the length of time that the bladder can be ischemic under different conditions in people with obstruction?

- Can we develop non-invasive blood flow measurement tools in humans?

- Are antioxidant therapies effective in the treatment of obstructive bladder disease?

Genomics and Proteomics Technologies

The widespread use of microarray technology has been hampered by several factors that should be addressed. These barriers are as follows:

- The absence of a biotechnology center that produces cDNA arrays based on bladder libraries. None of the biotechnology centers recently funded by the National Institutes of Health is related to urology.

- Technical barriers that range from poor experimental design to lack of equipment and expertise to perform experiments and analyze data. Investigators of lower urinary tract dysfunction should be trained in all aspects of microarray analysis, and a separate training module should be devoted to bioinformatics and data analysis.

- The costs of using microarray technology are virtually insurmountable for the average investigator. Therefore, initial support for development of Biotechnology Centers in Urology with abilities to synthesize oligonucleotides and print arrays and perform hybridization will ensure that the scientific community could use this technology at significantly reduced cost. By providing these services at reduced cost, the centers will not only provide inexpensive microarray service to the urologic community, but also act as a stimulus for commercial vendors to lower their price barriers.

Questions to ask in genomics and proteomics research of the lower urinary tract are as follows:

- What is expressed differently in the nerves supplying the pelvic viscera?

- Is there a genetic predisposition that leads to voiding disorders?

Novel Therapies, Technologies, and Gene Therapy

Novel therapies and technologies include the promotion of re-innervation, gene delivery, devices for neurocontrol, regulation of the development of new blood vessels (angiogenesis), and novel drug delivery systems targeted at nerve transmission that is selective to the urinary tract.

One example of lower urinary tract gene therapy is that which could be used for stress incontinence. The concept of gene therapy strategies for stress incontinence is to build up the deficient urethral sphincter. To achieve this, tissue engineering or cell-based *ex vivo* gene therapy appears to be more logical than conventional viral vector gene therapy.

According to one study, muscle-derived, cell-based tissue engineering may have several advantages over the current treatment for urinary incontinence—collagen injection. The tissue engineering technique derives cells from the incontinence patient and then injects those cells back into the patient (autologous cell transplantation). The advantages of this technique are as follows:

- Transplanted cells will not cause an immune system or allergic reaction and, therefore, will survive longer than injected collagen derived from cows

- Transplanted cells can serve as a natural bulking agent when transplanted into the bladder and urethra

- Transplanted cells form muscle fibers that become innervated into the host muscle where they serve as a blocking agent and are physiologically capable of improving bladder (detrusor) muscle contractility

This study demonstrated three facts in the emerging field of urologic tissue engineering:

- The feasibility of injecting cells derived from skeletal muscle into the urethal sphincter

- The feasibility of gene transfer to the bladder and urethra

- The greater persistence of injected collogen derived from a patient's muscle versus injected bovine collagen

Unique Neurotransmission Principles

Neurotransmission principles unique to the lower urinary tract are relevant to the development of (1) drugs and therapies specifically designed for the lower urinary tract (i.e., identification of neurotransmitter pairing) and (2) effective agents that act on the central nervous system circuits of the lower urinary tract. Although important and likely to reveal useful therapeutic targets, most commercial activity is focused on unique neurotransmission principles; therefore, this area did not rank as highly as an area likely to yield rapid progress. Nonetheless, the following basic questions are relevant:

- How do nerves function differently in the bladder from nerves in other areas?

- How does this affect function—differentially?

Research Requirements

Research requirements are as follows:

- Loan forgiveness is essential to recruit physician investigators.

- Stable increased funding targeted to these areas is needed to attract young and seasoned investigators to the field.

- Centralized resources for genomic and proteomic research efforts will accelerate progress.

- Increased interaction and co-sponsorship with other institutes at NIH (i.e., the National Institute of Neurological Disorders and Stroke, the National Institute on Aging, and the National Heart, Lung, and Blood Institute) will foster synergy and efficiency.

Patricia Francis

Neurogenic Bladder, Multiple Sclerosis

Patricia Francis is a woman of many interests who has had significant success over a long career as a graphic artist, photographer, editor, and naval historian. All of these pursuits have been sharply curtailed or diminished by the effects of multiple sclerosis (MS), an autoimmune disease that destroys the myelin sheath protecting certain nerve fibers. She cannot use her hands very well and walks with great difficulty. She has trouble manipulating her cameras and equipment. An avid gardener, known throughout her community as the "Flower Lady" for the bouquets she delivers and the plant seeds she shares, Pat has unfortunately had to restrict this activity as well.

Once her ability to draw was compromised, Francis began work on a history of naval aviators who flew during the Korean War and in later military conflicts. However, the limited use of her hands has caused her to have problems with this project as well.

"Like Matisse, I've had to find different ways of making art," she says.

Francis began her own heroic struggle almost 15 years ago, at the age of 50, when she noticed that she was experiencing "increasing fatigue, weakness, and flu-like or lancinating nerve and muscle pain" that occurred at least three to four days a week and was associated with periods of physical activity. The physical limitations and pain continued undiagnosed until eight years ago, when she suffered a head injury from an automobile accident. Brain imaging studies taken as a result of the accident showed some abnormalities that in retrospect were indicative of multiple sclerosis.

Three more years passed before physicians could conclusively tell her she had MS. "As strange as it sounds, I was relieved and grateful to hear that there was a disease process at work," she says. "I knew something was wrong and had been wrong

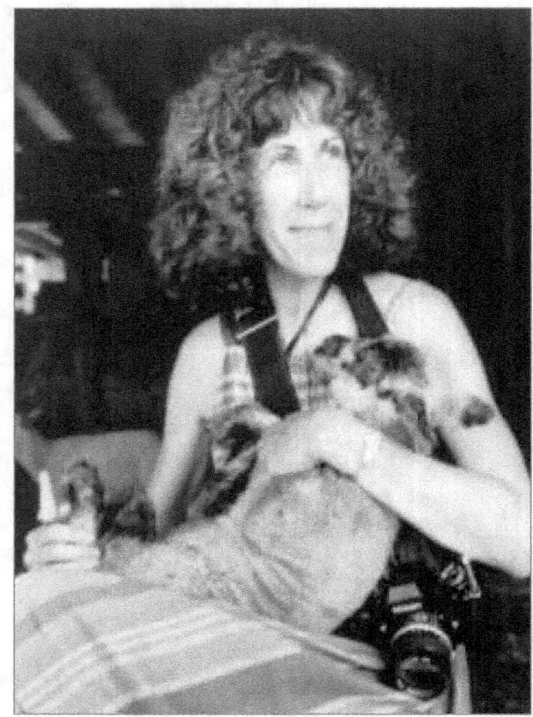

for many years, but I thought the diagnosis wouldn't be determined until I was autopsied. Now I could hope to find somebody who might be able to help me deal with the pain and other manifestations of the disease." By the time she was diagnosed, the nerve damage to her urinary tract caused by MS was so extensive that Francis lost significant sensation in her bladder and could no longer tell when it was becoming full.

In a neurogenic bladder, nerves that carry messages to the bladder muscle do not work properly. Francis experiences leakage of urine because the bladder muscle has lost tone, but she also experiences urinary retention because nerves do not relay the message that its time to let go. Urine that stays too long in the bladder can lead to a urinary tract infection, which could spread to the kidneys. It could also lead to reflux of urine into the ureters and kidneys, a condition that can cause kidney damage.

"I don't know when I have to urinate," Francis says. "When I'm out in public, this is especially hard. I feel a great sense of relief when I've been able to reach a bathroom without an accident." The problem is especially difficult because she walks with the assistance of two leg braces and a cane.

To lessen the severity of incontinence, Francis does preventive bladder training. She sees a physical therapist and does Kegel exercises to strengthen the muscles of the pelvic floor, using an electronic device to give her feedback on how well she is doing. Kegel exercises involve contracting and raising the pelvic floor muscles.

Francis also schedules when she voids. Before she leaves the house, she goes to the bathroom, and when she arrives at her destination, she goes again. "Either my bladder is not holding much, or it's unstable and making me go frequently," she says. "Because of this, traveling even a moderate distance is no longer an option. Rest stops are too far apart."

When Francis' bladder becomes full or releases urine, she has a great deal of cramping pain. The cramping disturbs her sleep, Francis says, which adds to the problem of nighttime voiding, a common occurrence in people with a neurogenic bladder. Sometimes she even dreams she is urinating and awakens with a start. These problems have placed her in a double bind. The urinary symptoms exacerbate the MS symptoms by causing her to not get enough rest, which would reduce her muscle pain.

"My body requires restorative sleep, not the kind of sleep that one gets with sleep medications," Francis says. "When I tried to take them, I felt even more tired and was unable to think effectively."

Francis struggles to keep a balance in her life between the activities she loves and the physical realities of her illnesses. She limits her fluids at night and when she leaves home. She limits the time she spends at the computer and the trips she takes beyond the borders of her home. She limits physical exertion. She has given up most of the artwork and the gardening that provided so much pleasure in the past.

Francis and her husband have also experienced the financial limitations of a chronic illness. "This is an expensive illness, and insurance doesn't pay for a lot of things I need," Francis says. "You have to juggle costs and decide what is more important to buy."

Although limits have become an integral part of her life, any conversation with her reveals an important truth. This is a woman who will not limit her creative ideas. She will make the adjustments, much as Matisse did, and like Matisse she will work despite the pain.

"My choice is to function as if I were a zombie or to be productive, so I deal with the pain by working," says Francis, explaining that she relegates the pain to the status of background noise. "I don't take medications during the day unless I can't stand it. When it seems to be getting worse, it's important to short circuit pain rather than wait until it's really bad."

When night comes, it's a different story. Pain medications provide welcome relief. "At night, it's hard to make bladder pain and the 'bee-stinging' pain of MS background noise," she explains. "By the end of the day, one is tired of coping with pain."

SECTION B COMMON CLINICAL CONDITIONS

Bladder disease in its many forms affects the health and well being of millions of Americans. Some diseases of the bladder—bladder cancer, posterior urethral valves, and cloacal exstrophy, to name a few—are life-threatening, requiring surgery, other therapies, and long-term follow-up. Other diseases such as interstitial cystitis, vesicoureteral reflux, and urinary tract infections may cause more widespread problems in the upper urinary tract—the kidneys—or in other body systems. Loss of normal organ function and the resulting chronic health problems that are debilitating, painful, and costly in terms of personal finances, emotional health, and productivity are frequent outcomes of these complications.

Seemingly less serious, chronic conditions such as urinary incontinence may also have potentially severe effects. Incontinence with urinary leakage may appear to those without the problem to be a condition of the elderly that people, especially women, learn to live with as they grow older. In fact, urinary incontinence may affect people of all ages and creates burdens similar to other chronic health problems. These burdens are magnified by the social stigma attached to the leakage of urine.

Other bladder conditions are caused by diseases that develop first in other systems, such as diabetes, a disease of the endocrine system, and multiple sclerosis, a disease of the nervous system. While these diseases may only involve the urinary tract secondarily, in some situations the primary symptoms may be urinary incontinence or other symptoms of bladder or urinary tract dysfunction.

Although basic scientific research on the lower urinary tract will increase our knowledge of how the bladder functions, this basic knowledge needs to be translated into active clinical research that will take what has been learned in the laboratory to the patients who suffer from these diseases and who volunteer for a studies that will eventually benefit other patients.

The Bladder Research Progress Review Group has selected high-impact bladder conditions on which to focus this report and has recommended research priorities. The high-impact conditions include the following: problems of the developing genitourinary tract in children; urologic conditions of maturation and aging; bladder outlet obstruction; interstitial cystitis; urinary tract infections; effects of diabetes; urinary incontinence; and cancer.

CHAPTER 5

PROBLEMS OF THE DEVELOPING GENITOURINARY TRACT IN CHILDREN

Common Clinical Conditions

DID YOU KNOW?

→ Genitourinary birth defects are the most common congenital abnormalities in newborns.

→ Approximately one out of every 5,000 to 8,000 male infants are born with posterior urethral valves, which have immediate life-threatening consequences.

→ Vesicoureteral reflux affects an estimated 1 percent to 2 percent of children and is the most common cause of kidney failure in children.

→ About one in 5,000 infants are born with spina bifida, the most common primary cause of neurogenic bladder dysfunction in children.

Summary and Recommendations

Normal bladder function is a critical part of human development. Abnormal bladder development can have profound consequences such as constant urinary leakage and, ultimately, deterioration of kidney function. An improved understanding of lower urinary tract development will not only facilitate the treatment of childhood voiding disorders, but also provide insight into adult disorders. Many bladder pathologies that affect adults—obstruction and loss of nerve supply, for example—recapitulate fetal events.

The Bladder Research Progress Review Group made an extensive and comprehensive review of this research area and developed the following recommendations for future research:

→ Investigate the mechanisms of lower urinary tract development and dysfunction at the molecular, genetic, and cellular levels to identify the causes of neurogenic bladders, voiding problems, and problems causing obstruction to urination

→ Develop better treatment for these disorders

→ Determine the epidemiology and confounding factors related to bladder diseases and develop a means of evaluating prospectively and longitudinally the risk factors related to problems such as urinary tract infections, vesicoureteral reflux, daytime wetting, enuresis, and hydronephrosis.

Specific recommendations for each developmental condition are located at the end of this chapter.

Background

During normal bladder development, dramatic changes occur that are critical for normal bladder function. In the fetus, the bladder is initially an extension of the ureters, and it acts as a conduit for urine, which then flows out of the fetus' body through the urachus and into amniotic fluid. Only with time does the bladder develop a storage function. The initial stages of this function begin in the older fetus as it develops reflex emptying. This process continues after birth and throughout the next few years of normal human aging. In time, the child develops voluntary sensory control of urination. Thus, normal voluntary continence with normal bladder storage and emptying takes complex coordination between the bladder and the urethra.

In the normal state, the bladder is a supple, distensible organ. Urine is transported to the bladder from the kidneys via the ureters. The bladder's function is to store urine at a constant low pressure, then empty completely at socially acceptable intervals. This low-pressure storage concept can be described as bladder elasticity. Abnormal excessive bladder contractions caused by disease, may cause the bladder to lose elasticity, changing to a stiff-walled, high-pressure storage chamber.

Abnormal development, injury, disease, or the aging process itself can interrupt or reverse this normal bladder developmental path, causing problems of inadequate storage or emptying, that is, involuntary voiding or incontinence, as well as serious consequences ranging from frequency and urgency to urinary leakage, vesicoureteral reflux, infections, stones, and, ultimately, deterioration of kidney function requiring dialysis.

One example of an anatomic developmental problem that occurs in the embryo is bladder exstrophy. In infants born with bladder exstrophy, there is a gap in the anterior wall of the bladder and the abdominal wall located in front of it exposes the bladder's posterior wall.

Abnormal embryonic development in other body systems such as the nervous system can also cause an anatomically normal bladder to develop abnormally. This occurs, for example, when the spinal cord, especially the lower part, develops abnormally. Several conditions can result from this, depending on the extent of the abnormal development, but these conditions are generally known as myelodysplasia. Later in life, diseases that affect the nervous system such as diabetes and Parkinson's disease, spinal cord injuries, and aging also have an impact on the lower urinary tract.

Genitourinary birth defects are the most common congenital abnormalities in newborns. In children, abnormal bladder function secondary to abnormal development occurs frequently. Common problems include spinal cord defects (spina bifida), congenital and acquired bladder outlet obstruction (posterior urethral valves, ectopic ureteroceles, dysfunctional voiding), and congenital anatomic anomalies (bladder exstrophy, imperforate anus, prune belly syndrome, and ureteral ectopia). A significant number of children who are born with these defects, which are described below, will have morbidity directly related to their bladder function.

Epidemiology

From a socioeconomic point of view, abnormal development of the lower part of the spinal cord or myelodysplasia constitutes a significant health problem in the United States. The incidence of spina bifida, a form of myelodysplasia, is reported to be approximately 1 per 5,000 live births. Approximately 70 percent of people with myelodysplasia have decreased bladder elasticity that is clinically significant.

Posterior urethral valves occur only in males. They are membranous folds that develop within the posterior (prostatic) urethra, and it is estimated that they occur in one out of every 5,000 to 8,000 births of male infants. Because these folds or valves obstruct the outflow of urine, approximately 30 percent of infants with valves have a clinically significant decrease in bladder elasticity. Congenital bladder outlet obstruction has immediate life-threatening consequences as well as long-term consequences on kidney and bladder function. There does not appear to be any known ethnic or familial predisposition toward the development of posterior urethral valves.

Vesicoureteral reflux, the abnormal retrograde flow of bladder urine into the upper urinary tract as the result of an incompetent junction between the ureter and the bladder, affects approximately 1 percent to 2 percent of children. Vesicoureteral reflux can result in severe infection and kidney failure and is a common cause of the latter in children. In children who do not have urologic symptoms or a history of infection, the incidence of vesicoureteral reflux is estimated to be less than 1 percent. In children with a history of symptomatic urinary tract infection, the incidence of this condition is estimated to range from 20 percent to 50 percent.

Enuresis or bedwetting, another persistent and pervasive problem, might reflect abnormal bladder development as well. More common in boys than in girls, enuresis affects 5 million to 7 million children between the ages of 6 and 18. The incidence varies in different societies, but in five-year-old children in the United States, the incidence is about 15 percent to 20 percent. About 1 percent to 2 percent of older adolescents have nocturnal enuresis. After the age of six, childhood bed-wetting or enuresis becomes a very important problem for the child and the parents. In addition, some evidence indicates that children with enuresis might be predisposed to future bladder problems as adults.

Daytime urinary incontinence, nocturnal enuresis, and dysfunctional voiding affect an estimated 5 percent of families with children. Approximately 15 percent to 20 percent of children are incontinent during the day at age 5, 5 percent at age 10, and 1 percent above age 15.

Developmental Problems

Developmental problems affecting the bladder in fetuses, newborns, children, and adolescents, may be grouped into the following categories:

- Abnormal or injured nerve development: myelodysplasia, neurogenic bladder

- Associated anatomic abnormality: posterior urethral valves, vesicoureteral reflux, ureteroceles, ectopic ureters

- Unclear causes: nocturnal enuresis; dysfunctional voiding; non-neurogenic, neurogenic bladder

- Incomplete or abnormal anatomic development: exstrophy and its variants, prune belly syndrome, imperforate anus, and cloacal abnormalities

These problems are described in the sections that follow.

Myelodysplasia and neurogenic bladder—Myelodysplasia is an abnormality in the development of the spinal cord, especially the lower part of the cord. Neurogenic bladder is bladder dysfunction that originates in or is caused by the nervous system or nerve impulses. In children, spina bifida, a type of myelodysplasia, is the most common primary cause of neurogenic bladder dysfunction. Second siblings in the same family have a 2 percent to 5 percent risk of being born with the same disorder.

Spina bifida arises from a defect in the formation of the neural tube. The cause of this defect is uncertain, but various teratogens such as alcohol and zinc, as well as some medications such as valproic acid, have been implicated. Recent evidence has suggested that a deficient maternal intake of folic acid is associated with the development of spina bifida and that supplementation may reduce the chances of acquiring such birth defects seven-fold.

About 95 percent of children with spina bifida have abnormal innervation of the bladder. Because of increased bladder pressure and the potential for vesicoureteral reflux, obstruction, and infection, children with spina bifida are at risk for kidney damage unless nerve and bladder abnormalities are recognized early and intervention is prompt.

Children with spina bifida have long-term problems with bladder control and need clean, intermittent catheterization several times a day in combination with anticholinergic drugs. This regimen is inadequate for many children, who often require multiple surgical interventions to allow adequate urinary storage. Surgical interventions may include bladder augmentation or replacement with portions of intestine and bladder neck procedures to improve continence. However, none of these treatments is ideal, and many children suffer from the consequences of inadequate and improper urinary storage. Complications may include bacteriuria, stones, continual leakage, and, in the most severe cases, deterioration of renal function related to persistent high bladder pressures.

Major short-term care costs include the costs of surgery, if it is possible, to close the vertebral arches through which the spinal cord and meninges protrude, hospitalization, and imaging evaluation. Long-term health care costs include costs for follow-up visits, surgery, urodynamic measurement, chronic medication, diapers, caretakers, lost work for parents, multidisciplinary health care teams, and ultimately, lost work for the person with this problem as he or she becomes an adult.

Vesicoureteral reflux—Vesicoureteral reflux, the abnormal retrograde flow of urine already in the bladder into the upper urinary tract, is the result of an incompetent junction between the ureter and the bladder. Vesicoureteral reflux and its associated recurrent UTIs are the most common causes of renal scarring in children and may cause severe renal dysfunction. In children with reflux nephropathy or renal scarring from vesicoureteral reflux and infection, hypertension and progressive renal dysfunction may occur even if the reflux resolves.

Reflux is the most common cause of kidney failure in children. It is often detected in children who have had recurrent urinary tract infections (UTIs) or an unexplained, recurrent febrile illness. Infections are often severe and kidney failure frequently results. In children with a history of symptomatic urinary tract infection, the incidence has been estimated to range from 20 percent to 50 percent. In those who do not have urologic symptoms or a history of infection, the incidence is less than 1 percent. Hydronephrosis, dilation of the kidney pelvis and calyces, is a secondary outcome of reflux, and it can be detected by prenatal ultrasound. However, most infants born with vesicoureteral reflux alone are asymptomatic at birth.

Risk factors for vesicoureteral reflux are as follows:

- *Age* — Reflux is most common in very young children and incidence declines with age.

- *Race* — Reflux is more common in fair-skinned children. It is significantly less prevalent in black children and in children of Mediterranean origin when compared with white children. White girls have been reported to have 10 times the incidence as black girls.

- *Sibling predisposition* — Reflux occurs in approximately 40 percent of the siblings of children with known reflux. Younger siblings are at greatest risk. In many of these children, there may be no documented history of symptomatic infections. For this reason, most pediatric urologists and nephrologists advocate routine screening of siblings of children with known reflux.

- *Sex* — Because of the epidemiology of UTI in children, boys and girls may present with reflux at different ages. In the neonatal period, UTIs are more common in uncircumcised boys than in girls; therefore, many more boys will be diagnosed with reflux. After the first year of life, the incidence of UTIs becomes much higher in girls than in boys; therefore, most school-age children diagnosed with reflux are girls.

An increased understanding of the pathologic mechanisms and the natural history of reflux have led to improvements in both medical and surgical approaches to treating this condition. Effective treatment greatly depends on early detection and the institution of antibiotic prophylaxis. The primary goal in both medical and surgical management is to prevent development of pyelonephritis, an inflammation and infection of the kidney, and the formation of scarring. Close follow-up and periodic reevaluations are necessary for all children with this problem. When indicated, surgical correction of reflux has been shown to be safe and effective.

Short-term costs for vesicoureteral reflux include the costs of evaluation and imaging. Long-term costs are for medications, surgery, imaging evaluation, renal insufficiency, hypertension, and transplantation.

Posterior urethral valves—Posterior urethral valves are the most common congenital cause of bladder outlet obstruction and one of the most common urologic emergencies that occur in fetuses and newborns. Incidence has been estimated to be one per 5,000 to 8,000 male births. The immediate survival of the infant with posterior valves depends on early recognition and stabilization of the acute metabolic abnormalities that result from obstruction.

Occurring only in male infants, posterior urethral valves are membranous folds within the posterior (prostatic) urethra. These folds obstruct the outflow of urine. The presence of valves becomes evident in a wide spectrum of clinical symptoms, depending on the degree of obstruction that developed in the fetus. Urethral valves may be detected before birth by prenatal ultrasound examination or after birth. Prenatal diagnosis of posterior urethral valves has provided pediatricians and pediatric urologists with an opportunity to initiate treatment immediately after birth.

Signs and symptoms of posterior urethral valves in a newborn that has not been diagnosed prenatally are as follows:

- Respiratory distress

- Presence of microorganisms in the blood and tissues (sepsis)

- Abnormal levels of urea and other nitrogenous substances in the blood plasma (azotemia)

- Abdominal distention

- Bladder dysfunction

Congenital bladder outlet obstruction can be life threatening, and it has long-term consequences on kidney and bladder function.

Approximately one-third of all children with valves will have significant lower urinary tract dysfunction manifested most commonly by urinary incontinence. In a small but significant number of children, bladder dysfunction may be so severe as to lead to further deterioration of renal function.

Definitive relief of the obstructing valves can be achieved surgically, using several techniques. Long-term medical management includes a frequent timed voiding regimen to reduce urinary residual and stasis, which can lead to infection; anticholinergic medications to treat those children who manifest low-capacity, hyper-reflexic bladders; clean intermittent catheterization for poor emptying of the bladder; antibiotic prophylaxis for persistence of vesicoureteral reflux; and treatment of renal insufficiency, if needed (some children with valves continue to have deterioration of kidney function resulting in chronic renal insufficiency).

Renal insufficiency can lead to a variety of metabolic abnormalities and growth retardation. In cases where surgical and medical therapies fail, it may be necessary to surgically augment the bladder capacity to achieve urinary continence and preserve renal function. Bladder augmentation using gastrointestinal segments produces its own metabolic complications depending on the intestinal segment used. Long-term follow up in these children is necessary because they may also be at significant risk of malignancy.

Health care costs for children with posterior urethral valves are disproportionately high when compared with the number of infants affected with this condition. Long-term costs are high because children with poor outcomes such as kidney failure need chronic care.

Voiding dysfunction and daytime incontinence—The term voiding dysfunction in childhood means a dysfunction of the lower urinary tract that does not have a recognized organic cause (e.g., neurological disease, injury, or congenital malformation). Although the term voiding dysfunction is more accurate, it is often used interchangeably with the term "bladder dysfunction." In general, voiding dysfunction is a disturbance in the coordination between the bladder muscle and the external sphincter activity. It can take many forms, including the inability to voluntarily start or to stop voiding, poor bladder emptying, incontinence, and high pressures in the bladder.

Normal lower urinary tract function includes storage of urine at low pressures (made possible by an accommodating, low-pressure bladder and a closed sphincter) and voluntary emptying (including not only a voluntary bladder contraction, but also an involuntary sphincteric relaxation just before bladder contraction). Because older children can control their external sphincter more easily than their bladder muscle, they can more easily stop urination than start it. Contraction of the external sphincter is subconscious and normal during bladder filling, but it is pathologic during bladder contraction or voiding. In the worst of these cases, this can cause lower (and upper) urinary tract deterioration.

Daytime urinary incontinence is the involuntary leakage of urine in a child older than five years of age (the age at which a normally healthy child in our society should have acquired daytime continence). This particular age how-

ever depends on the culture of the family. For example, in some Asian families continence is expected between ages two and three.

Daytime urinary incontinence, nocturnal enuresis, and dysfunctional voiding affect an estimated 5 percent of families with children. Approximately 15 percent to 20 percent of children are incontinent during the day at age 5, 5 percent at age 10, and 1 percent above age 15. About 80 percent of all of these children are incontinent only at night.

By the age of four, most children with a normal and healthy development can manage both the bladder maturity and social skills required to stay dry during the day. The prevalence of urinary incontinence (UI) in children has not been well studied mainly because the definition of voiding dysfunction or functional incontinence is unclear. However, the following points are known:

- Of all children with a wetting problem, 10 percent will only have symptoms by day, 75 percent only by night, and 15 percent by both day and night.

- About 15 percent of five-year-old children have UI, mostly at night.

- Studies in children just starting school (six to seven years of age) have shown that 3.1 percent of the girls and 2.1 percent of the boys had an episode of daytime wetting at least once a week. Most of these children had urinary urgency (82 percent of the girls and 74 percent of the boys).

- For reasons that are not understood, there is also a difference in prevalence depending on whether the child lives in colder (2.5 percent) or hotter areas (1 percent).

- The spontaneous cure rate for daytime wetting is similar to that for nocturnal enuresis (about 14 percent of children will improve without treatment each year).

- A strong association exists between bladder dysfunction and bacteriuria. However, it is not known whether the bacteria cause the bladder dysfunction first or vice versa (it is likely that bladder dysfunction causes an increased rate of bacteriuria). Probably, both are true, and this often leads to a "vicious cycle."

- The diagnosis of a urinary tract infection (UTI) should not be overlooked because in children symptoms are often systemic (e.g., fever and failure to thrive), rather than localized in the urinary tract.

- Bladder dysfunction is also commonly associated with bowel dysfunction. The anal sphincter, the external urinary sphincter, and the pelvic floor muscles constitute an integrated unit. Treatment of chronic constipation and encopresis can result in complete resolution of bladder symptoms.

- A higher incidence of bed-wetting occurs when daytime wetting is present. However, a corollary of this is that daytime wetting or frequency without concomitant nighttime incontinence or nighttime voiding (nocturia) is most likely not organic.

Many studies have noted psychiatric disturbances associated with dysfunctional voiding. However, it is difficult to differentiate whether psychological factors or social pressures are the primary reason for the voiding problem, or whether the incontinence has led to psychosocial problems. In a condition with severe social consequences, separating cause from effect is difficult. Psychosocial or psychiatric help should only be the primary focus in unusual cases (e.g., sexual abuse).

A child with dysfunctional voiding may have a functional obstruction where the bladder muscle joins the sphincter (detrusor-sphincter dyssynergia) and, therefore, high pressure within the bladder at voiding. Recognizing the voiding dysfunction that presents along with vesicoureteral reflux is important because surgical correction of the reflux will often not change the child's voiding habits and, therefore, only part of the problem will be solved.

Urinary incontinence in children can be primary or secondary. Primary incontinence means that the child has never been dry. Secondary incontinence means that the child has been dry for at least six months and then starts to wet again. A history of secondary incontinence is of greater concern to clinicians because more consideration must be given to factors that might bring on this problem (e.g., infection, neurological abnormalities, or sexual abuse).

Many different varieties of voiding dysfunction exist, and they manifest different symptoms. While some forms may account for rare episodes of urinary leakage (giggle incontinence) in children, severe forms may cause urinary retention or such poor voiding (e.g., non-neurogenic neurogenic bladder or Hinman's syndrome) that bladder and kidney function are impaired. The causes and reasons for the different symptoms and signs are unclear.

Enuresis—Enuresis has been recognized for millennia, and it affects virtually all cultures. Defined as the persistence of inappropriate voiding of urine beyond the age of anticipated control, enuresis can occur both during the day and at night (diurnal) or at night only (nocturnal). Depending somewhat on the age of the child, about 15 percent of nocturnal enuretic children are also wet during the day. In a few, enuresis occurs only during the day.

Enuresis is more common in boys than in girls. In the United States, enuresis affects 5 million to 7 million children between the ages of 6 and 18. After the age of six, childhood bed-wetting becomes an important problem for the child and the parents.

Enuresis Possible Causes
• *Genetics*
• *Maturational delay*
• *Sleep disorders*
• *Psychological factors*
• *Urinary tract infection*
• *Nocturnal polyuria*

Enuresis can be categorized as either primary or secondary, depending on the child's history. Primary enuresis is designated if the child has always been wet, whereas the term secondary enuresis is used if the child has had a dry period of at least a month before wetting again. About 20 percent of children with nocturnal enuresis can be classified as secondary. Concern about the new onset of enuresis often encourages unnecessary investigation. The causes and treatments of enuresis vary considerably.

Nocturnal enuresis is a symptom (as opposed to a disease) and, as such, is likely to have many different causes. Furthermore, these factors are not mutually exclusive, and children may have a complex interrelationship of explanations. Possible causal factors are genetics, maturational delay, sleep disorders, psychological factors, urinary tract infection (UTI), and nocturnal polyuria.

In many cases, the cause of enuresis remains uncertain because an extensive evaluation is invasive and not generally cost-effective. Therapy in a given child is often prescribed without regard to the specific etiology.

Enuresis has a strong genetic component. The incidence is 77 percent among children whose mother and father both had enuresis, 44 percent if one parent had enuresis, and 15 percent if neither parent had enuresis. Monozygotic twins (identical twins) have twice the concordance than dizygotic twins (fraternal twins).

Costs of enuresis treatment vary according to the therapy and supplies. Therapy includes positive reinforcement methods; anticholinergic and antidepressant drugs; desmopressin acetate, a synthetic antidiuretic hormone administered at night via nasal spray; conditioning techniques using an alarm that goes off when urine connects with the circuit; avoidance of allergenic foods; and hypnotherapy and psychotherapy, which are not considered appropriate for the average child.

Exstrophy-epispadias complex—Exstrophy-epispadias complex is an all-encompassing term for a spectrum of congenital anomalies of the bladder and urethra that range from epispadias, a malformation in male infants in which the urethra opens on the dorsal aspect of the penis, to cloacal exstrophy, a complex of severe abdominal anomalies that can affect both male and female infants. Exstrophy-epispadias complex occurs in one infant per 30,000 to 40,000. Within this spectrum of anomalies, classic bladder exstrophy occurs in 60 percent, epispadias (all forms) in 30 percent, and complex cloacal exstrophy and other variants in 10 percent.

In the embryo, persistence of the cloacal membrane after the fourth week of gestation prevents the lateral mesoderm from migrating medially. Once the membrane disappears by the ninth week, the posterior wall of the bladder is exposed to the outside, with the umbilicus adjacent to the bladder wall.

In the most common form of primary epispadias—penopubic—the urethral opening (meatus) is located where the base of the penis joins the lower abdominal wall. Other variations may exist including a very mild form of dorsal glanular epispadias, where the urethral meatus is located at the back of the head of the penis.

The most severe form of epispadias, cloacal exstrophy, occurs in the early stages of embryonic development. In the developing embryo, the urorectal septum normally forms and divides the cloaca, a chamber into which the hindgut and allantois empty, into anterior and posterior compartments. However, when an abnormally large cloacal membrane perforates before the cloaca is divided, an exstrophied bladder separated by an exstrophied ileocecal bowel area results. Children born with this condition usually have two everted bladder units separated by an everted segment of the intestine, generally the cecum, which has a blind end. At birth, the exposed bladder and urethra are obvious malformations. Exposure of the bladder results in bacterial colonization, thickening of the bladder, and resultant fibrosis, which replaces muscle and reduces the bladder's elasticity. Up to 66 percent of the children with cloacal exstrophy have problems in the upper urinary tract as well.

Once the bladder has been surgically closed, vesicoureteral reflux occurs in most children as a result of the abnormal placement of the ureters and the lack of muscular backing by the bladder. Inguinal hernias are common (both direct and indirect), especially in boys. The testes are normally descended in most cases. Some children may have rectal prolapse (10 percent to 20 percent) because of muscle weakness in the pelvic floor.

In girls, the clitoris is divided on both sides of the urethra; the vagina is tilted anteriorly and may often be narrowed. Despite this, girls are potentially fertile. In boys, the penis usually is significantly rotated and shortened. The corporal bodies of the penis are separate (unlike the normal penis in which the corpora communicate) and diverge to attach to the inferior rami of the pubis, which are rotated laterally and anteriorly. Thus, osteotomy, performed on the pubic bone to restore normal distance at the symphysis (the cartilaginous joint that unites the two sides of the pubis), results in further shortening of the already stubby penis.

Significant problems are associated with this anomaly, including herniation of the abdominal organs into the umbilical sac (omphalocele) and numerous gastrointestinal anomalies, including malrotation, duplication, duodenal atresia (absence of a normal opening or lumen), and Meckel's diverticulum, (a remnant of the embryonic yolk sac that forms a blind pouch in the intestine). Significant genitourinary anomalies, including separate bladder halves and cleft genitalia, are also associated with this condition.

Newborn males are often gender converted to female as a result of inadequate genital development and the poor prognosis for developing a normal male phenotype. In the past, children with the most severe and rare form (incidence of 1:200,000 live births) of the exstrophy-epispadias complex were usually left to die. With modern surgical techniques and a multidisciplinary approach to their care, children with this complex disorder can achieve acceptable lifestyles.

Recently, a staged approach to closure has been found to provide adequate drainage of kidneys and to enhance the potential for continence after reconstruction. The three phases of the staged approach are as follows: (1) primary bladder closure, performed during the newborn period, (2) epispadias closure, performed between six months and one year of age, and (3) bladder neck reconstruction and ureteral re-implantation.

With the current staged approach, continence rates of up to 50 percent and 60 percent have been reported, although this varies among treatment centers and surgeons. In most children who remain incontinent after the staged procedures, the bladder capacity is to blame. Surgical bladder augmentation or creation of a bladder reservoir using bowel can be performed to solve this problem. In some children, the bladder outlet is weak, and placement of an artificial urinary sphincter or urethral augmentation with collagen or Teflon injection may be beneficial.

> **Stages of Exstrophy Closure**
>
> **Stage 1:** *Primary bladder closure, performed during the newborn period to convert the extrophied bladder to an epispadias*
>
> **Stage 2:** *Epispadias closure, performed between six months and one year of age*
>
> **Stage 3:** *Bladder neck reconstruction and ureteral re-implantation*

Renal deterioration is prevented if bladder pressures remain relatively low and if the child remains on antibacterial prophylaxis because of reflux. In children with more severe forms of exstrophy who may require urinary diversion (e.g., connecting the ureters to an abdominal stoma or opening), upper tract damage can occur, and it varies according to the type of diversion.

Imperforate anus—Imperforate anus comprises a spectrum of anomalies involving the anus and rectum; these anomalies range from simple anal fistula to complex cloacal malformations involving multiple organ systems.

By the eighth week of gestation, the primitive hindgut in the embryo becomes separated into the rectum and the urogenital sinus by the descending urorectal membrane. Incomplete migration or fusion of the membrane may result in persistent communication between the rectum and the urogenital sinus—a fistula—as well as malformations of the pelvic musculature (sphincter).

Anorectal anomalies can be divided into high, intermediate, or low defects based on the level of the fistula between the rectum and the urinary tract or on the degree of malformation or absence of the rectum. Most children with high lesions will require a colostomy to temporarily divert fecal material until a more distal repair can be accomplished. In lower or more minor lesions, a minor reconstruction of the posterior portion of the rectum and anus may accomplish the job without having to resort to a colostomy. Until lower urinary tract anomalies are ruled out or reconstructed, children are placed on prophylactic antibiotics to avoid sepsis, the presence of pathogens in the blood.

Associated anomalies of imperforate anus are seen in up to 50 percent of cases and urologic involvement in 26 percent to 50 percent. Generally, the more severe the defect, that is, the higher the connection between the rectum and urethra or between the rectum and vagina, the higher the incidence of associated anomalies.

Factors contributing to morbidity in these children are related mainly to genitourinary anomalies, spinal (especially sacral) anomalies, other malformations, and the quality of bowel and urinary sphincters.

Prune belly syndrome—Prune belly syndrome (PBS) is sometimes referred to as Eagle-Barrett, triad, or mesenchymal dysplasia syndrome. The incidence of these syndromes ranges from one in 35,000 live births to one in 50,000 live births, with most cases occurring in boys and only 3 percent to 5 percent in girls. Prune belly syndrome has three major pathologic anomalies, although other coexisting orthopedic, pulmonary, and cardiac anomalies have been noted as well: (1) deficient or absent abdominal wall musculature; (2) various ureteral, bladder, and urethral abnormalities involving marked dilatation; and (3) bilateral undescended testes.

The definitive origin of prune belly syndrome remains controversial, but two theories predominate:

Obstructive theory—Severe bladder outlet obstruction existed early in gestation and was subsequently relieved after irreversible damage had occurred. Obstruction resulted in bladder distention, ureteral dilation, and hydronephrosis, as well as atrophy of the abdominal wall muscles by the increased pressure and interference with the blood supply. However, most children with prune belly syndrome lack anatomic obstruction at the time of birth.

Mesodermal defect theory—A primary defect in mesenchymal development occurred early in gestation.

Imperforate Anus Associated Anomalies

- *Spinal malformations*

- *VACTERRL syndrome (Vertebral, Anal, Cardiovascular Tracheal, Esophageal, Radial, Renal, and Limb abnormalities)*

- *Genitourinary anomalies*

Clinical manifestations of prune belly syndrome are as follows:

- **Kidneys:** Kidney abnormalities are the major determinants of survival, with a 20 percent chance of stillbirth or death in the neonatal period from renal dysplasia and the associated pulmonary hypoplasia. An additional 30 percent of children will develop urosepsis or renal failure or both in the first two years of life.

- **Ureters:** Severely dilated and tortuous, the ureters are most severely affected at the lower end and appear to have patchy areas of fibrosis. Vesicoureteral reflux is present in 75 percent of these children. Although their radiographic appearance is alarming, drainage is generally adequate.

- **Bladder:** The bladder is generally capacious, smooth-walled, and irregularly thick, without a meshwork of fibers (trabeculation). Often, a remnant of the urachus (the urinary outlet in the fetus that connects the bladder to the umbilicus) or a diverticulum (an out pouching of the intestinal wall) creates an hourglass configuration. Functionally, children with these bladders exhibit a diminished sensation of fullness and have a large capacity with poor contractility, decreased voiding pressures, and, thus, a poor ability to empty.

- **Prostate gland and posterior urethra:** The prostatic urethra is elongated and characteristically tapers to the membranous region, which gives rise to the typical radiographic appearance of a triangular posterior urethra.

- **Anterior urethra:** Although the urethra is most often normal in this syndrome, both urethral atresia (absence of a urethral opening or of a patent urethral lumen) and megalourethra (dilation of the urethra) can be seen.

- **Testicles:** Cryptorchidism (failure of both or one of the testes to descend) is seen universally in boys with prune belly syndrome, the gonads characteristically being found high in the abdomen. Histologically, the testes are markedly abnormal, thus rendering patients infertile.

> **Prune Belly Syndrome Major Anomalies**
>
> - *Deficiency or absence of abdominal wall musculature*
>
> - *Ureteral, bladder, and urethral anomalies, manifested in most cases by marked dilation*
>
> - *Bilateral undescended testes*

- **Abdominal musculature:** The most characteristic manifestation of prune belly syndrome is the wrinkled, "prune-like" skin of the abdomen in the newborn infant. Skeletal muscle underdevelopment is seen in all three layers of the abdominal wall muscles. Complications are surprisingly minimal. The inability to sit up directly from the supine position may delay the onset of walking, but it rarely affects normal physical activity.

- **Other associated anomalies:** Other anomalies are found in more than 65 percent of children, the most common being cardiopulmonary and gastrointestinal, and include orthopedic and developmental problems as well. Pulmonary abnormalities range in severity, with the most significant arising in cases where the mother has an insufficient amount of amniotic fluid (oligohydramnios). Children who survive the neonatal period usually have no associated pulmonary problems.

Prenatal ultrasound is capable of detecting abnormal urinary tract dilation as early as 14 weeks gestation. However, differentiating prune belly syndrome from other causes of urinary tract dilation is difficult. In the presence of oligohydramnios, prenatal intervention has been advocated to decompress the dilated bladder and restore the amniotic fluid volume. Although prenatal intervention may improve pulmonary function, its ability to improve kidney function is uncertain.

Children with severe forms of prune belly syndrome usually do not survive the neonatal period; however, for the few who do survive, urinary diversion is often recommended to provide optimal urinary drainage.

Moderately affected children with PBS usually are treated medically unless infection persists despite antibiotic prophylaxis, renal growth is inadequate, or renal function is decreasing. In these cases the urinary tract is reconstructed with ureteral tailoring and correction of reflux to reduce stasis. Reconstruction of the abdominal wall and repair of the undescended testicle(s) (orchidopexy) are often performed simultaneously.

Mildly affected children have good renal function; therefore, surgical intervention is usually not necessary. However, life-long antimicrobial prophylaxis is often instituted. Repair of the undescended testicle(s) may be delayed until such time as any other reconstructive procedures may become necessary or at about six months.

Abnormalities of bladder drainage are the principal source of problems in childhood, and they may lead to renal deterioration. Pyelonephritis or renal deterioration may prompt a re-implantation and, perhaps, tailoring of the ureters to improve drainage and prevent reflux. However, these procedures are complicated because of poor peristaltic movement of the ureters and the abnormal bladder into which they are reimplanted. Because of persistent stasis of urine postoperatively, nearly all children with this condition are maintained on lifelong antibacterial prophylaxis.

Adequate drainage can be obtained with clean intermittent catheterization, but this can be difficult because children with prune belly syndrome have normal urethral sensation and some have urethral anomalies. For this reason, a continent abdominal stoma, an opening to the surface of the body, may be useful.

Persons who survive infancy with mildly impaired kidney function may develop kidney failure as a result of chronic pyelonephritis and damage to nerves from reflux (reflux nephropathy). Clean, intermittent self-catheterization to alleviate chronic retention should be performed. Kidney transplantation can be performed successfully. Early intra-abdominal repair of testicles is warranted in boys with prune belly syndrome because repair in infancy allows placement of the testicles into the scrotum without division of the spermatic vessels, which may not be possible later in life. Although likely to be infertile, these children may benefit from advances in fertility techniques in the future. Major reconstruction of the abdominal wall can be done at the same time as orchiopexy.

Ureteroceles—A ureterocele is a cystic dilatation of the terminal intravesical segment of the ureter. Ureteroceles are discovered in 1 in 500 autopsy cases. They occur four to seven times more frequently in females and are more common in white children. Ureteroceles are bilateral in 10 percent of cases. Eighty percent of cases are associated with the upper pole of a duplex system, and 60 percent have an orifice located ectopically in the urethra.

Ureteroceles are classified as being either *intravesical* (within the bladder) or *ectopic* (some portion extends beyond the bladder neck). Other terms commonly encountered include *stenotic* (intravesical with a small orifice), *sphincteric* (ectopic with the orifice within the urethral sphincter), *sphinctero-stenotic* (same as sphincteric with a stenotic orifice), and *cecoureterocele* (some part extends beyond the bladder neck, but the orifice is in the bladder).

In the first few months of life, children with a uretero-cele are most commonly diagnosed by a clinician who is seeing them for symptoms of a urinary tract infection. Some ureteroceles are detected incidentally on antenatal ultrasonography. Some children may have a palpable abdominal mass secondary to an obstructed kidney. Although urethral obstruction is rare, the most common cause of urethral obstruction in girls is urethral prolapse of a ureterocele.

Diagnostic tests for ureterocele are abdominal ultra-sonography; intravenous urography (IVU); voiding cystourethrography (VCUG), which is performed in all children with this problem; renal scan, which will determine the relative function of all the renal segments; and cystoscopy.

The type of treatment of a ureterocele depends on the type and the mode of presentation. Most children will require surgery, which ranges from endoscopic incision to complete open reconstruction. If the child presents with sepsis, secondary to obstruction, then immediate drainage of the kidney is necessary. Often, endoscopic incision of the ureterocele is the first step.

Ectopic ureters—The ureters normally insert into the bladder wall in the trigone region of the bladder. When a ureter inserts below this region, it is said to be *ectopic*. The ectopic ureteral opening is always along the pathway of normal development of the mesonephric system. Thus, in boys, it may lie in the bladder neck, prostate (to the level of the ejaculatory duct orifice), or even along the course of the male genital system, including the epididymis. In girls, the orifice may lie in the bladder neck, urethra, vagina, or, rarely, in the cervix and uterus.

Ectopic ureters occur more commonly in girls than in boys (ratio of 6 to 1). Approximately 70 percent of ectopic ureters are associated with complete ureteral duplication. Boys are more likely than girls to have single

system ectopia. Associated with this condition, is a high incidence of abnormal tissue development in the segment of the kidney parenchy-ma that is drained by the ectopic ureter. Also, the incidence of contralateral duplication is as high as 80 percent.

> **Facts about Ectopic Ureters**
>
> - *More common in girls than boys (a ratio of 6:1)*
>
> - *Usually discovered during a doctor's visit for UTI*
>
> - *Often associated with abnormal tissue develop-ment in the kidney*
>
> - *Requires surgery or bladder reconstruction or replacement.*

In boys, ectopic ureters are usually discovered during an evaluation for urinary tract infections. If the ectopic ureter enters the genital ducts, epididymoorchitis, a simultaneous inflammation of the epididymis and testis, is possible. Boys never present with incontinence because the ectopic ureter is always inserted above the external urethral sphincter.

In infancy, girls usually present at examination with a urinary tract infection. However, older girls tend to present with incontinence. This is usually described by the parent as the child always being wet even though she has normal voiding habits, or the child becoming more wet when sitting on the parent's lap (urine pooling in the dilated ureter or vagina). If the ectopic ureter is located outside the urethra and the kidney has developed abnormal tissue, some children may have pyonephrosis, pus in the kidney that distends the pelvis and calyces.

Diagnostic tests for ectopic ureter are abdominal ultrasonography; intravenous urography (IVU); voiding cystourethrogram (VCUG); dye tests, if the sonogram, IVU, and VCUG fail to establish the diagnosis; diuretic renography, an important test to assess upper pole renal function before surgery; and cystoscopy, which can be helpful in identifying the ureteral orifice within the urethra.

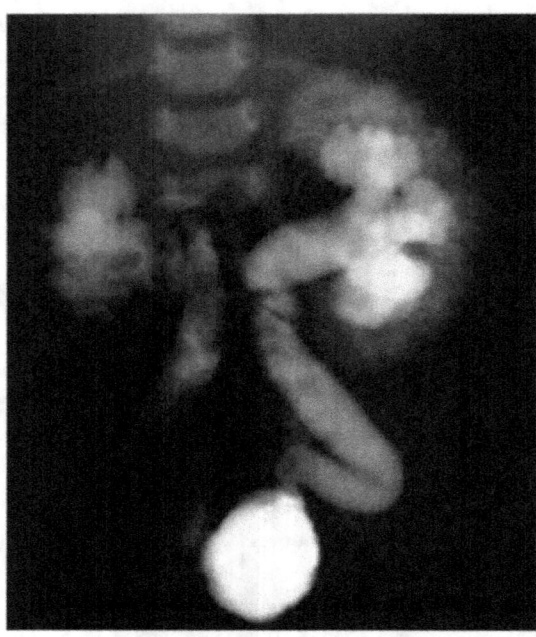

A voiding cystourethrogram of an infant girl with a febrile urinary tract infection shows bilateral grade 4 vesicoureteral reflux. On voiding, the urine backs up from the bladder (bottom) into the ureter and kidney (upper right). *(Photo Credit: Digital Urology Journal, Pediatric Uroradiology Rounds, Reflux and Intrarenal Reflux, http://www.duj.com. Copyright Digital Urology Journal)*

The type of surgical treatment of ectopic ureter depends on whether or not it presents in a duplex or single system. At times when the bladder is totally dysfunctional, bladder reconstruction or replacement may be needed. This is usually done using intestinal segments. Urinary tract reconstruction may also be required in children with bladder dysfunction that is secondary to spinal cord injuries, myelomeningocele (protrusion of the spinal cord and it membranes through a defect in the vertebral column), posterior urethral valves, cloacal anomalies, exstrophy, and other bladder abnormalities.

The ideal bladder augmentation or bladder substitution technique has been elusive. Current methods incorporate gastrointestinal segments into the urinary tract and result in many complications. These complications include calculi (stones), electrolyte imbalance, mucus production, bone demineralization, and perforations. None of the current reconstructive or replacement techniques is ideal.

Current Research

Research on the developmental anomalies of the lower urinary tract has been woefully lacking. Currently, only five studies of lower urinary tract development are sponsored by the National Institutes of Health (NIH). Much more needs to be done to determine the causes of these devastating conditions, which engender much suffering and debilitation for children and their families. New research studies are needed to build on the current state of knowledge determined by previous research. These studies should focus on

- Nitric oxide protective mechanism of fetal bladder function

- Developmental aspects of calcium mediation of contraction. Past studies have shown that the fetal bladder is more dependent on extracellular calcium for mediating contraction, thus indicating a significant difference between the bladders of fetuses and newborns and the bladders of adults in their sensitivity to calcium channel blocking agents and potassium channel openers

- Coordination between vascularization of the developing bladder's smooth muscle elements and the contractile function of the smooth muscle. (Since ischemia may be a major factor in fetal bladder dysfunction, this is an important focus area for future research.)

- Genetic characterization of bladder problems

- Bioengineering of bladder tissue

- Pharmacologic manipulation of continence with relation to bladder innervation

- Mesenchymal epithelial signaling in development and disease

- Fetal and developmental bladder physiology

- Defining bladder markers (characteristics or factors by which a cell or molecule can be recognized and identified) such as uroplakin

- Epithelium-stroma interactions

- Fetal sheep model of bladder development

- Fetal surgery

- Tissue engineering

Research Opportunities

Research opportunities exist in many areas that have been virtually ignored by research projects. Research studies are needed to

- Characterize and define the epithelium

- Characterize and define the stroma and the smooth muscle cells

- Determine the epithelial-mesenchymal interactions in the normal state and during disease

- Identify growth factors

- Explain the process involved in bladder wound healing

- Develop new techniques and materials for bladder replacement

- Determine the abnormal cellular signaling involved in developmental anomalies

- Determine the genes involved in pediatric bladder disease

- Develop *in vitro* and *in vivo* models for bladder development with biomaterials

- Determine the efficacy and benefit of fetal surgery for bladder abnormalities

- Continue to develop fetal models of normal, obstructive, and neurologic injury

- Create a bank of human DNA samples (tissue samples)

- Apply genomic research to variants using microarrays to determine polymorphisms related to variants

- Work with human and mouse genome initiatives

- Create animal models

- Understand the pathophysiology of bladder and urinary tract muscle developmental response in fetus, neonate, and growth through adolescence associated with non-obstructive and obstructive hydronephrosis

- Develop new fetal diagnosis and monitoring technologies for bladder and urinary tract developmental anomalies

- Explore the potential use of pharmacotherapy in the fetus

- Investigate the use of drugs to treat an uncoordinated sphincter

- Determine the consequences of long-term pediatric drug use

- Explore gender differences in pharmacological sensitivity

- Define the role of estrogen receptors in regulating lower urinary tract function

- Determine differences in response to pharmacological agents among fetuses and neonates

- Institute preventive measures at childhood such as healthy bladder habits and pelvic floor muscle programs that can prevent future bladder dysfunction

Research Requirements

More investigators are needed in the field; therefore, fellowships should be established in all areas that promote studies in bladder function. To advance this goal, the Bladder Research Progress Review Group (BRPRG) made the following suggestions:

- Provide academic fellowship training support

- Establish awards

- Offer loan forgiveness

- Make the grant award system less cumbersome

- Establish a means of time-sensitive interaction with the NIH

- Recognize the clinical applicability and limitations of current models (animal versus human, female versus male)

- Establish curriculum on urinary incontinence in medical schools

- Create tissue banks and urine storage for future studies on children with bladder dysfunctions.

- Encourage research that studies the spectrum of bladder dysfunctions across the lifespan, from pediatrics to geriatrics. In this respect, the BRPRG recommends that the NIH encourage new investigators in this field under the auspices of established bladder investigators.

Recommendations for Specific Conditions

The BPRG made the following specific research recommendations for each developmental condition described in this chapter and for other related disorders.

Myelodysplasia, Spina Bifida

- Explore the means to prevent spina bifida through diet, fetal treatment, or C-section

- Explore the efficacy of neonatal versus delayed treatment of bladder dysfunction

- Address the psychosocial effects of spina bifida and bladder dysfunction

- Investigate the long-term outcome of bladder dysfunction in persons with spina bifida

- Investigate the effects of early pharmacological therapy

- Determine the feasibility of re-innervation of the bladder

- Identify the genes that are involved and determine how reversible they are, either genetically or pharmacologically

Vesicoureteral Reflux

- Develop non-invasive diagnostic techniques

- Determine the risk of stopping antibiotic prophylaxis

- Determine long-term outcomes and fetal and maternal risk

- Establish genetic markers

- Develop endoscopic surgical approaches and injectable materials

Posterior Urethral Valves

- Develop non-invasive diagnostic techniques

- Develop fetal intervention techniques for renal and bladder function

- Determine long-term outcomes

- Identify genetic markers

- Develop endoscopic surgical approaches

- Develop new drug therapies

Urinary Incontinence. Dysfunctional Voiding. and Enuresis

- Determine the mechanisms of normal voiding

- Identify genetic markers

- Develop new pharmacologic interventions

- Establish awareness and education programs

Exstrophy-Epispadias Complex. Imperforate Anus. Prune Belly Syndrome

- Develop better diagnostic techniques

- Identify genetic markers

- Develop new pharmacologic interventions

- Establish awareness and education programs

- Improve surgical techniques

Ureterocele. Ectopic Ureters

- Develop diagnostic techniques

- Identify genetic markers

- Develop new pharmacologic intervention

- Establish awareness and education programs

- Determine long-term outcomes

- Define obstruction

- Determine who needs treatment

- Identify the need for antibiotic prophylaxis

- Develop new surgical techniques

- Establish embryological studies

Colin Golliver

Cloacal and Bladder Exstrophy

Colin Golliver and his twin brother, Sean, were born seven and a half weeks prematurely with serious problems that even an ultrasound did not entirely anticipate. Sean had two large hernias that caused him a great deal of pain, but Colin had cloacal and bladder exstrophy, one of the most serious birth defects a newborn could face.

"When my doctor first saw Colin, he couldn't tell if he was a boy or girl," says Susan Golliver, the twins' mother. "He had an exposed bladder that seeped urine, his abdominal organs herniated into the umbilical cord, his penis was in two parts, and his testicles were inside his body." In addition, his mother said, Colin's large bowel was in two parts and his spinal cord was tethered," that is, strands of it were attached to his tailbone, a problem that would cause him to develop nerve damage resulting in numbness or loss of feeling in his legs as he grew.

Cloacal and bladder exstrophy is a rare and complex congenital malformation that occurs in the embryo during the early weeks of pregnancy when tissues that form organs are developing. It requires skilled medical and surgical care for years after birth. Infants born with this malformation have abdominal organs located outside the abdomen, an open bladder, a rectum that communicates with the bladder, absence of the rectum's normal anal opening, spinal defects, and a pelvic bone separated in the front. In girls, the vagina is often absent and the clitoris is split in two; in boys, the penis and scrotum are divided into two halves. The cause of cloacal exstrophy is unknown, and in many parts of the world, boys who are born with it are often surgically converted to girls.

Immediately after birth, Colin was transferred to the pediatric intensive care unit of Children's Hospital in Tulsa, Oklahoma, an hour and a half from his home. Three days later, he had the first of many surgeries to correct his problems. Because his upper colon was not connected to the rectum, surgeons

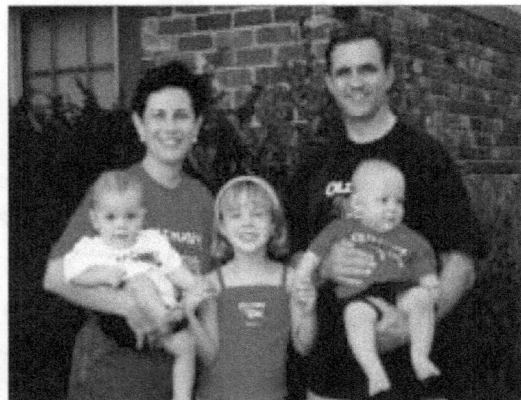

The Golliver Family *(Colin shown on left)*

connected it the surface of his abdomen, where his bowel movements could now be eliminated into a bag that would be glued to the skin surrounding the stoma or abdominal-intestinal opening. The surgery went well and in November, Colin re-entered the hospital for his next surgery—freeing his spinal cord from his tailbone. This surgery also went well, but his parents and physicians would not know how this problem would affect his ability to use his legs until he developed further.

The following December, after receiving two hormone injections to enlarge the two halves of his penis so that they could be joined, Colin had his third major surgery, which lasted 14 hours. Surgeons closed the bladder, repaired his hernias, surgically constructed an anus, brought his undescended testicles to the outside of his body, and joined the two portions of his penis. Fixator pins were also inserted into the two sections of Colin's pelvis to join the pubic bones.

Colin's post-operative period was as complicated as his surgery. Because of the fixator pins, he had to lie on his back for several weeks, making normal things that parents do for their babies—bathing, feeding, burping, diaper changing, and cuddling, for example—extremely difficult. In addition, Colin's mother also emptied her son's colostomy bag and provided skin care for the area around the stoma. "We couldn't hold Colin, but we talked to him a lot," says Golliver, who expressed her milk and fed him with a bottle. At times, she even bent over him and nursed him. By the end of January 2002, six weeks after surgery, Colin was doing well. His repaired bladder, which surgeons cautioned often doesn't stay sealed, was functioning normally, and he was urinating on his own. However, Susan had to intermittently catheterize him to be sure his bladder was emptying.

In February, after a long winter of providing physical and emotional care to her three children, Susan Golliver became seriously depressed. At this time, surgeons were anticipating the next surgery—attachment of the two portions of Colin's bowel and repair of the stoma. To prepare her son's colon for the surgery, Golliver had to gradually dilate the stoma several times a day with metal rods that increase in diameter. It was a procedure that caused Colin to scream in pain and his mother to crumble.

"One day I woke up and thought, 'What have I gotten myself into? I just can't handle this anymore,'" Golliver says. "I had been strong for months because of the surgeries. I had been going on adrenaline for so long."

Golliver attributes the depression to her disappointment that she could no longer continue to nurse her sons and to the subsequent hormonal changes that were occurring as she weaned them. Stress, lack of sleep, and the demands of her husband's job, which was threatened by his company's financial difficulties, were also contributing factors.

"My body just couldn't keep up with the demand," Golliver explains. "I had had months of interrupted sleep, where I couldn't get more than two to three hours at a time." She also rarely left her house. Once she stopped nursing the twins, a decision she made reluctantly, her husband Tom, who was working long hours during the day, was able to share the night shift with her. With more sleep, her depression began to lift. Relatives were also able to pitch in even more than they had previously, including babysitting so that Golliver could run errands.

In early April, Colin had his fourth surgery. The two portions of his colon were successfully connected making a colostomy unnecessary. In May, at the age of nine months, a time when most children are crawling, as is his brother Sean, Colin was still having difficulty sitting in his high chair, but he was trying to move about the floor by rolling, according to his mother. "The pediatrician is not concerned," she says, "because he has full range of motion." Colin is receiving physical therapy to strengthen his muscles, and his mother believes that before long he will be able to follow Sean's lead.

Surgery to relocate the urethral opening from the backside of Colin's penis to the normal position at its tip is scheduled next. Surgeons are also considering re-implanting a ureter into the bladder because Colin has had two bladder infections and vesicoureteral reflux, a condition in which urine backs up into the ureter(s) and kidney(s), where it can cause scarring and impair function. Reflux is a potentially devastating condition for all children but particularly for Colin because he has only one kidney. Constipation may also become a problem, even though it has not happened so far. If it should become chronic, his mother says further surgery will be necessary to keep the bowel patent.

"It's been a hard journey," says Golliver, "but Colin is a blessing to our family. He has taught us to face each day with hope, faith, and empathy for others. Through all of his trials, he has been such a peaceful baby. God definitely gave him a sweet disposition to deal with his pain." Golliver also pays tribute to Colin's surgeons, who she says treat him with respect and dignity. "They are like an extended family to us, providing us with not only their medical expertise, but also great emotional support."

Colin's sister, Lauren, as well as her parents, are still puzzling about why Colin developed this problem. "I told [Lauren] that no one knows, but maybe she will become a doctor when she grows up and figure it out," Golliver says. "This type of birth defect happens between the 8th and 12th weeks of pregnancy, a time when most people don't even know they're pregnant. Maybe in the future, scientists will find a way to prevent it or do something to correct it [before the child is born].'

Timothy Hawkins

Vesicoureteral Reflux

At the age of 18, Timothy Hawkins doesn't remember much about the pain and discomfort he experienced as a little boy, when he was frequently sick. His mother, Mary Pat, says he suppresses that memory because "he went through a lot." What Tim does remember is as follows: Going to the bathroom and seeing "all these lumps of things in my urine." Having high fevers and going in to the doctor's office and hospital for numerous tests—"ultrasounds and a VCUG" or voiding cystourethrogram, a diagnostic test that involves threading a catheter through the urethra, filling the bladder to maximum capacity with a radiographic dye solution, and following the flow of urine on x-ray as the child voids. Taking antibiotics every day between the ages of three and five to prevent kidney infection and to preserve kidney function. Going into the hospital with his parents for surgery when he was five years old for the removal of his right kidney. And having bad dreams after surgery that he thinks were caused by "the pain killers I took."

"My right kidney was deteriorating because I had reflux," Tim says. "The urine backed up into both my kidneys, but the right one was worse. When I was in kindergarten the right kidney had to be removed." Vesicoureteral reflux is the abnormal flow of urine from the bladder back into the ureter(s) and kidney(s). It is the most common cause of kidney failure in children and is usually diagnosed when a urinary tract infection or UTI occurs.

About one-third of children with UTI have reflux, which can occur from primary or secondary causes. Primary reflux occurs during fetal development when the tunnel in the bladder wall where the ureter inserts fails to grow long enough, thereby preventing the valve that forms at that juncture from closing properly. This permits backflow of urine and bacteria into the ureter(s) and even the kidney(s). Secondary reflux occurs as the result of conditions such as posterior urethral valves (see profile of Hayden Gantz, Chapter 7), which obstruct the urethra, or bladder infection that causes swelling.

Tim's mother has more vivid memories of those years. She describes Tim's fevers, which were also caused by ear infections, as "raging" and frequent, and remembers putting him in a tub of tepid water to bring them down. She remembers her son telling her at the age of three that "sometimes poop comes out from where I pee" and the horror she felt when she saw dark lumps in the bottom of the toilet bowl after he urinated standing up. She remembers the anger and frustration she felt toward Tim's pediatrician when he told her over the phone that she was probably over-reacting and that she should give her son cranberry juice.

"Neither Tim's pediatrician nor the emergency room physicians took a urinalysis to see if the problem was caused by a urinary tract infection, a sign of reflux," Mary Pat says. "A urinalysis is now done routinely when a child has a high fever."

She also remembers her father, a physician, urging her to ask Tim's doctor to perform an ultrasound to visualize Tim's urinary tract, and she remembers making an urgent phone call to her sister-in-law, a radiologist, to ask her to find someone who would do this when Tim's physician said it was unnecessary.

Mary Pat and her husband Jim soon decided that they needed to consult a pediatric urologist at a major medical center. "She placed Tim on continuous antibiotic therapy to see if his kidneys would heal," Mary Pat explains. Antibiotic therapy usually corrects secondary reflux caused by infection, and it prevents further damage if the cause is primary, that is, genetic.

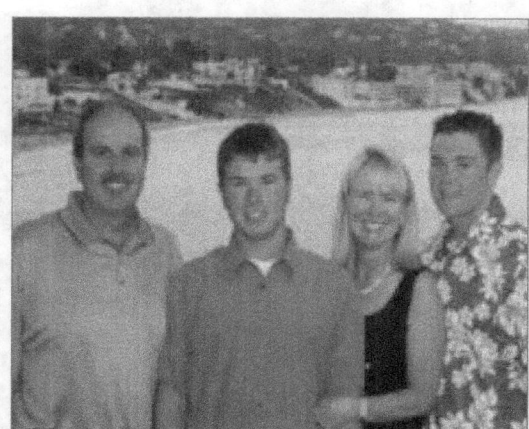

The Hawkins Family (*Tim, second from left*)

faster, he decided it was time to drop out. In high school, he took up golf, which he has grown to love, and has played on his school team. "I sometime wish I could play football, though, but that's not an option," he adds.

Tim has been monitored with ultrasounds periodically to see if his remaining kidney is growing. "It grows larger to make up for the kidney that was removed," he explains. He recently had an MRI to check on scarring in that kidney. "Everyone has a little scarring. It can occur when you hold back going to the bathroom," he says. "But I'm more susceptible to it because of the reflux."

Many children also outgrow reflux. During a period of "watchful waiting" to see if this would occur, Tim was monitored at intervals with urinalyses, ultrasounds, and VCUGs. However, when he was five years old, it became obvious that the right kidney was not going to heal, and it had to be removed.

By age nine, Tim's urologist determined that his reflux was primary and that it had not improved in the left ureter. Re-implantation of the ureter was now necessary because his urologist feared that in time it would cause further damage to his remaining kidney. The surgery involved lengthening the canal in the bladder wall where the left ureter inserts and then re-implanting the ureter.

Tim describes his life since his surgery as "fairly normal." He graduated from high school last June and this fall will go to Santa Clara University in California. Although he has not been able to play contact sports since his first surgery because of the risk of injury to his remaining kidney, he has found other outlets for his interest in sports. He played Little League baseball for a few years, learning to bat left handed so that if he were hit by a wild pitch, the side that doesn't have a kidney would absorb the impact. But when the pitches got

Recently, one of Tim's younger cousins was discovered to have reflux after he developed bladder control problems and side pain. At the age of 6, the cousin's ureter was reimplanted. Because of the familial implications, Tim has begun to think about what a genetic disease will mean for his children.

"My doctor says that some reflux is genetic and there's a good chance that my kids would have the same problem with reflux," he says. "Maybe by doing research, doctors could test my kids before they develop problems or even before they're born so that they don't develop scarring and high blood pressure or lose a kidney."

CHAPTER 6

UROLOGIC DISEASE IN MATURATION AND AGING

Common Clinical Conditions

DID YOU KNOW?

→ During aging, the urethra deteriorates in many people, and urethral pressure declines 1 percent per year.

→ Aging causes a decline in the bladder's ability to contract but also a dramatic increase in the prevalence of involuntary contractions.

→ Aging causes a decline in bladder capacity.

→ Prostate enlargement and outlet obstruction are common and costly problems in aging men.

→ Urinary incontinence caused by changes in the urethra and bladder is a common and costly problem for aging women.

Summary and Recommendations

For reasons that are not well understood, the incidence and prevalence of urologic disease—especially urinary incontinence, benign prostatic hyperplasia (BPH), urinary tract infections, prostate cancer, and neurogenic bladder—increase with age. The aging process itself, even in the absence of disease, is likely a major contributor.

Unfortunately, little is known about the effects of age on the bladder and urethra. The dearth of human research in this area and the lack of accepted experimental models have hindered medical knowledge about the urologic problems of maturation and aging and limited prevention and treatment options as well. The little data that are available from clinical studies suggest that lower urinary tract function changes substantially with age. In women, urethral length and elasticity, as well as sphincter strength, seem to decline with age. In men, the prostate enlarges, although it is not known why there is variability in the degree of growth and its varied effects to bladder function on storage and emptying

After an extensive and comprehensive review of this research area, the Bladder Research Progress Review Group (BRPRG) has recommended that future research do the following:

➡ Investigate the developmental mechanisms and the disease mechanisms of the lower urinary tract at the molecular, genetic, and cellular levels to identify the causes of neurogenic bladders, voiding problems, and problems causing obstruction to urination and to develop better treatment for these disorders.

➡ Examine the aging urinary tract at the molecular and cellular levels and understand the causes of dysfunction.

➡ Establish clinical research programs that deal with the pathophysiology and management of the aging and dysfunctional urinary bladder and sphincter.

Specific studies related to each of these areas have been recommended by the BRPRG and are listed below:

➡ Developmental and Disease Mechanisms

- Genetic mechanisms

- Molecular and cell biology

- Developmental markers

- Stem cell and cell lineage studies

➡ Epidemiology and Genetics

- Longitudinal studies

- Prospective database

- Validated questionnaire

- Psychosocial factors

- Identification of developmental risk factors leading to adult lower urinary tract dysfunction

➡ Epigenetics

- Urinary tract infection

- Aging

- Clinical studies of normal older people coupled with basic science (molecular and cell biology)

- Relevant experimental models

Background

Lower urinary tract function changes substantially with age, according to some research studies on human subjects. In women, the length and elasticity of the urethra appears to decline with age, and sphincter strength seems to diminish. In men, the prostate appears to enlarge, although whether or not this is true in all men is unknown.

An improved understanding of the development of the lower urinary tract will provide greater insight into disorders brought on by maturation and aging and facilitate their prevention and treatment. Many adult bladder pathologies such as obstruction and loss of nerve supply recapitulate fetal events.

The Urethra and Urinary Incontinence

The urethra is the organ that provides closure of the lower urinary tract and prevents incontinence. Urinary incontinence (UI) is a remarkably common condition, particularly in women. The medical and work-related costs of urinary incontinence are estimated to be $26 billion dollars per year.

The two most influential urethral factors in urinary incontinence are urethral function and urethral support. Despite the high prevalence of UI, almost nothing is known about the factors involved in the growth and development of a proper urethra (or its support structures); how the urethra deteriorates with age; and how good function and support can be maintained throughout maturation and aging.

The urethra has a complex layered structure, including circular striated, longitudinal, and smooth muscle surrounding a specialized sealing core of blood vessels and mucosa. Once formed, the urethra deteriorates during the aging process. Urethral pressure declines 1 percent per year after adulthood. Early exploratory studies have indicated that striated muscle cell numbers in the urethra decline 2 percent per year; loss of smooth muscle has not been studied. This loss of striated muscle is twice as great as that found in other parts of the body, and the cellular and genetic factors for this accelerated loss are not known.

Perhaps the greatest human sexual dimorphisms exist in the urethra. Gaining insight into the development and physiology of the female urethra should lead to important improvements in understanding urinary incontinence and its treatment. For example, if the mechanisms for increased deterioration in the muscle within the urethra wall were known, preventive strategies might be sought and advice given to women to prevent this problem from developing.

Understanding why some women lose muscle must be based on an understanding of the cellular and genetic mechanisms that maintain normal muscle bulk. The effect of neural connections, growth factors, vascular supply, proper response to normal stresses, and the signals and genetics of these processes in the urethra deserve research attention equal to that in the bladder.

The signaling mechanisms that result in the proper orientation, integration, and maturation of the urethra's muscle layers are virtually unstudied. In addition to forming adequate quantities of smooth and striated muscle, the urethra must integrate with the abundant connective tissue in the sphincter to effect closure. Failure of these critical steps could lead to inadequate closure of the sphincter in the adult. Identification of the processes of urethral function and the genes that control them may explain the known familial aspect of urinary incontinence.

A second area important to continence concerns the levator ani muscle (the muscle that raises the pelvic floor) and the endopelvic fascia. Contraction of the levator ani muscle at the time of increased abdominal pressure plays an important role in maintaining urethral closure and integrity of this mechanism. Connective tissue supports of the urethra connect the muscles to the urethral support apparatus and provide strength to the urethra in maintaining continence.

Bladder Dysfunction

In both sexes, aging appears to cause a decline in the contractility of the bladder's detrusor muscle and a dramatic increase in the prevalence of involuntary detrusor contractions. Aging also appears to cause a decline in bladder capacity. Furthermore, the ultra-structure of the bladder muscle (detrusor) may change substantially with age. In the only study of this to date, aging was associated with an increase in the space between or among cells; a decrease in the density of normal smooth muscle junctions (adherens); and the appearance of junctions called protrusion or abutment junctions, which are not seen in younger people.

In the protrusion or abutment junctions in older people, the space between cells is significantly smaller than in normal smooth muscle junctions. Two other features of bladder muscle in younger people are also absent: (1) the abutting basement membranes that interpose central linear density and (2) the dense plaques normally present below the sarcolemma that anchor the converging ultramicroscopic threads of proteins that make up muscle fibrils (myofilaments). Such changes may reflect de-differentiation and may even set the stage for the emergence of involuntary bladder muscle contractions in the elderly.

A dramatic decrease also occurs in the number of cell caveolae, small pockets in cells that extend outside the cell wall; this phenomenon may mediate the decline in muscle contractility. Because these data, like the physiological data cited previously, are virtually all derived from small, cross-sectional studies, it is not clear how much this decrease in caveolae reflects the process of aging itself or the influence of cohort and secular effects (e.g., the number of pregnancies, the obstetrical practice). The impact of subclinical neurological disease has not been well addressed in studies, further limiting the ability to disentangle the effects of the aging process from other factors. Moreover, the cause of such changes—regardless of underlying associations—is completely unexplored.

The changes brought on by aging are virtually uninvestigated in other important areas as well. These areas include epithelial structure and function, bladder immune function, and changes in neural control stemming from changes in the neural axis from the cerebral cortex to the nerves that innervate the bladder.

Nighttime voiding or nocturia is another common problem faced by elderly men and women, and it is reported in approximately 80 percent of persons over age 75. Nocturia causes significant sleep deprivation and has been reported to be a cause of falls and hip fracture. Therefore, in addition to morbidity, it has a significant impact on quality of life and medical costs.

Besides developing abnormal bladder elasticity, older people can also develop poor bladder contractility secondary to muscle and nerve damage incurred by other illnesses associated with aging (e.g., diabetes). Secondary dysfunction causes significant morbidity. Damage incurred during surgery and possibly from aging of the musculature of the urinary bladder sphincter can also lead to significant morbidity from urinary incontinence.

Outlet Obstruction and Post-Prostatectomy Incontinence

As men age, the prostate enlarges. Obstruction of the bladder outlet is a common outcome that can affect bladder function and have a great economic impact on older men. Overactive bladder is also increasingly prevalent in aging men, as a consequence of obstruction, as a function of aging, or both.

A clinically significant decrease in bladder elasticity occurs in approximately 20 percent of men with benign prostatic hyperplasia (BPH). In the United States, about two in ten men with BPH will have prostate surgery for relief of obstruction; however, relief does not necessarily return the bladder to a normal state.

Prostate cancer starts to have an impact on men in their sixth decade of life and beyond. As more and more younger, healthy men undergo radical extirpation of the cancerous prostate, the incidence of post-prostatectomy urinary incontinence increases. These problems are serious and, although not life-threatening, have a dramatic impact on quality of life and overall medical costs.

The incidence of post-radical prostatectomy incontinence ranges from a low of 5 percent to a high of 60 percent, depending on whether the physician or the patient is reporting outcomes. Risk factors for this problem have been identified and include age and pre-existing bladder and sphincter dysfunction. Recent studies indicate that outcomes of surgical intervention for prostate cancer may depend on the specific techniques used to perform a radical prostatectomy.

[Editor's Note: Problems in the lower urinary tract that are related to aging such as obstruction of the bladder outlet and urinary incontinence will also be discussed in subsequent chapters with those titles.]

Current Research

Current research on bladder development includes studies on

- Laboratory models of human urothelium

- Amphibian bladder/No glucose transport model

- HOXA 13 regulation of vascular development

- Urogenital smooth muscle development

- Bladder remodeling and the role of growth factors

- Elastic microfibrils

The National Institute of Diabetes, Digestive, and Kidney Diseases (NIDDK) is currently funding studies of prostatitis, medical therapies of prostatic symptoms, urinary incontinence treatment, and interstitial cystitis treatment. Few individual grants are directed to the non-surgical management of urinary incontinence.

Major areas of recent advances in understanding the effects of maturation and aging are as follows:

- Genetic characterization of bladder problems

- Bioengineering of bladder tissue

- Pharmacologic manipulation of continence with relation to bladder innervation

- Mesenchymal epithelial signaling

- Definition of bladder markers (uroplakin)

- Epithelial/stroma interactions

- Fetal sheep model of bladder development

- Tissue engineering

- Neuromodulation of the sacral reflex arc to manage bladder dysfunction

Research Opportunities

Future research on the bladder and urethra during maturation and aging could focus on the following areas:

➡ Basic Mechanisms of Development and Aging

- Characterize and define urothelium, stroma, and smooth muscle cells

- Identify eptithelium-mesenchyme interactions in normal state and during disease

- Determine the relationship between growth factors and adhesion

- Explore the mechanisms of bladder wound healing

- Explore new techniques for bladder replacement

- Identify abnormal cellular signaling mechanisms

- Develop laboratory and human models for bladder development with biomaterials

➡ Genome Studies

- Identify and analyze genetic risk factors related to complications (e.g., renal insufficiency)

- Create a bank of human DNA samples

- Apply genomic research to variants using microarrays to determine polymorphisms related to variants

- Collaborate with human and mouse genome initiatives

- Create animal models

- Determine the effect of developmental bladder anomalies on an aging population (i.e., dysfunctional voiding effects on later incontinence in elderly people)

➡ Pharmacology Studies

- Identify sex differences in pharmacological sensitivity

- Determine the role of estrogen receptors in the regulation of lower urinary tract function

- Identify the differences among adults, including the elderly, in response to pharmacological agents

➡ Studies of Adult Women

- Gain insight into the development and physiology of the female urethra that will facilitate treatment and prevention of urinary incontinence (UI)

- Conduct longitudinal studies to understand the natural history of bladder diseases (i.e., the effect of early bladder disease on later bladder dysfunction)

- Elucidate opportunities for prevention (obstetric) of UI

- Explore opportunities for enhanced surveillance of hormonal effects and their influence on continence and incontinence

- Advance the knowledge of familial and genetic influence on continence mechanisms

- Investigate the relationship between UI and pelvic organ prolapse in women.

➡ Studies of Adult Men

- Determine and understand the risk factors that influence development of post-prostatectomy incontinence, incontinence that often develops after the prostate gland has been removed. A prospective study that considers good baseline information regarding continence status and other potential risk factors is necessary to understand and potentially to prevent the occurrence of incontinence after prostatectomy.

➡ Other Studies

- Create a longitudinal population database focusing on bladder function from childhood to aging. This database would pursue the prevalence and incidence of, and the risk factors for, various bladder dysfunctions (obstructed and irritative symptoms) and urinary incontinence. More specifically, the database would support a longitudinal study of children with specific bladder dysfunctions who would be monitored through childhood and adulthood. Ideally, data collection could include collection and preservation of tissue as well as documentation of symptoms and physical and urodynamic findings.

- Establish an animal model that could mimic the aging human bladder.

- Study the central nervous system's (CNS) control of human voiding in people with normal and abnormal bladder function. New technology such as magnetic resonance imaging (MRI) and positron emission tomography (PET) could be used to monitor control sites in the CNS

- Conduct studies to clarify the cause of nocturia in the elderly; this condition has a significant impact on their quality of life and on medical costs.

- Study childhood preventive measures such as healthy bladder habits and pelvic floor muscle programs

Research Requirements

Future research would benefit from the following areas:

Workforce

- Provide academic fellowship training support

- Establish awards

- Offer loan forgiveness

- Make the grant award system less cumbersome

Infrastructure

- Establish curriculum on urinary incontinence in medical schools

- Create tissue banks and urine storage for future studies on people with bladder dysfunctions

Implementation

- Develop a mechanism for time-sensitive interaction with NIH

- Recognize the clinical applicability and limitations of current models (animal versus human, female versus male)

- Encourage research that studies the spectrum of bladder dysfunctions across the lifespan, from childhood to old age

- Encourage new investigators in this field under the auspices of established bladder investigators

Alfred Arzberger

Post-Prostatectomy Incontinence

At the age of 68, after his prostate gland had been surgically removed because of cancer, Alfred Artzberger became incontinent. At first, surgeons thought the incontinence was the result of scar tissue forming in the upper urethra, where the surgery had been performed. Scar tissue interferes with the ability of the urinary sphincter, the circular muscle that controls the bladder outlet, to stay contracted. To correct the incontinence, surgeons dilated the scar tissue several times and then removed it, but Artzberger remained incontinent. Eventually his physicians concluded that during the delicate cancer surgery, a small section of the sphincter muscle had been excised along with the prostate. Artzberger's incontinence would be permanent.

"I leaked all the time," Artzberger says, "so I had to wear diapers. These were thin children's diapers—Huggies 5—which caused little to no discomfort." He continued to work as a sales executive and brought small plastic bags to work with him so that he could dispose of the diapers in the normal trash. He also informed his co-workers about his problem.

Eventually, Artzberger began to investigate possible solutions to his bladder problem. At the urging of his son, a physician, he consulted an expert on incontinence, who suggested a surgical implant of an artificial sphincter, a relatively new technology.

An artificial sphincter functions much like the biological one—it regulates the bladder's ability to store and empty urine. The implant consists of a cuff that fits around the bladder neck, a pressure-regulating balloon that is placed under the abdominal muscles and filled with liquid, and a control pump that inflates the cuff so that the urethra will close tightly. The control pump mechanism is usually placed in the scrotum for men and in the labia for women. The artificial sphincter stays contracted while the bladder fills

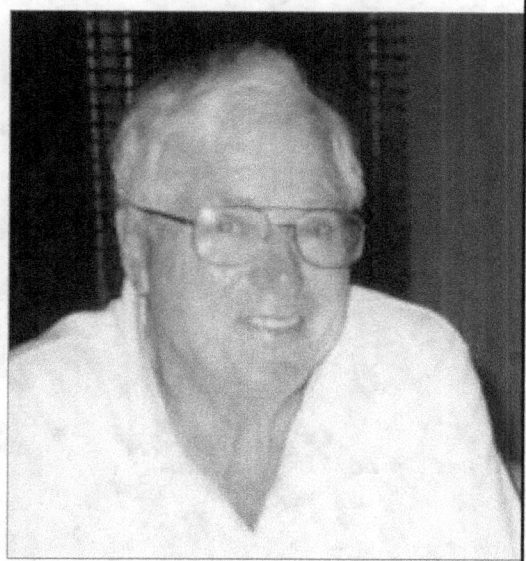

up. When Artzberger feels pressure from the full bladder, he goes to the bathroom as usual and relaxes the sphincter by pressing the valve in his scrotum.

"The bladder empties as near to normal as you can get," he says. "The only thing that's different is that after voiding, I have to wait about 20 seconds to allow the sphincter to close." Not everyone with an artificial sphincter implant has such positive results. Some patients experience urethral erosion—the eating away or inflammation of the surface layer of the urethra—or mechanical failure of the artificial sphincter, which must then be removed surgically. Infection is also an issue. "I've had tremendous success with the artificial sphincter," Artzberger says, "and I'm back to a normal life."

Five years after the implant, he continues to have good results and has had no adverse reactions. As a retiree at the age of 74, he plays tennis, enjoys golfing, does woodworking, and goes on vacations.

CHAPTER 7

BLADDER OUTLET OBSTRUCTION

Common Clinical Conditions

DID YOU KNOW?

→ Congenital bladder obstruction can cause irreversible bladder changes and life-threatening kidney problems.

→ Functional bladder obstruction — the loss of coordination between the bladder and its outlet—is a major problem for people with neurological disorders such as multiple sclerosis.

→ In most men, the prostate enlarges as they age, causing urinary frequency, urgency, nighttime voiding, and slow stream that can be not only annoying, but also life threatening.

Summary and Recommendations

Bladder outlet obstruction is a common condition, particularly in aging men, most of whom develop enlargement of the prostate gland or benign prostatic hyperplasia (BPH). Obstruction of the lower urinary tract may have several devastating consequences, including upper urinary tract deterioration with hydronephrosis (dilation of the pelvis and calices of one or both kidneys) and kidney failure. In children born with developmental bladder obstruction such as posterior ureteral valves (see Chapter 5, Problems of the Developmenting Genitourinary Tract in Children), obstruction causes not only irreversible bladder changes, but also life-threatening kidney changes.

For men with BPH, the more common and bothersome symptoms are those that have to do with voiding because they affect quality of life. BPH causes urinary frequency, urgency, slow stream, and nighttime voiding (nocturia), and it may also cause the bladder to empty incompletely. Incomplete bladder emptying is a predisposing factor for urinary tract infection (UTI), and total urinary retention follows in many cases.

Severe functional bladder obstruction also occurs in children with spina bifida, who can develop both severe urinary incontinence and kidney changes. People with neurological disorders such as spinal cord injury, multiple sclerosis, and myelomeningocele (protrusion of the spinal cord and its membranes through a defect in the vertebral column) often develop voiding dysfunction as well. Voiding dysfunction results from the loss of coordination between the bladder and its outlet and is characterized by functional bladder obstruction.

The Bladder Research Progress Review Group (BRPRG) made the following recommendations for future research efforts in bladder obstruction:

➡ Analyze the central and peripheral nervous system changes that contribute to voiding dysfunction in people with outlet obstruction, and thereby identify therapeutic interventions

➡ Determine the genomic and proteomic changes that underlie the alterations in the lower urinary tract that are produced by outlet obstruction, and thereby identify therapeutic targets

➡ Determine the impact of age on pathophysiology and treatment outcomes for obstruction

Background

Epidemiology

The prevalence of histological BPH increases steadily as a men age. Few men below age 30 have enlarged prostate glands, but 50 percent of men between the ages of 60 and 69 and 90 percent of men between ages 70 and 89 have BPH. Similarly, the prevalence of bladder outlet obstruction symptoms increases with advancing age. Moderate to severe symptoms are present in 18 percent of men ages 40 to 49 and in 56 percent of men ages 70 to 79. These symptoms increasingly interfere with quality of life as men age, causing them to seek treatments. The bladder's response to obstruction is the primary determinant of symptoms after BPH develops; therefore, emphasis on research in this area is crucial.

Although the highest incidence of bladder outlet obstruction is in the older male population, congenital bladder obstruction is far and away the more devastating problem because it results in life-threatening kidney changes in addition to irreversible bladder changes. The incidence of children born with urethral valves has been reported to be one out of every 5,000 to 8,000 male births. Of those children, up to 25 percent will go into end-stage kidney failure, requiring kidney dialysis and transplantation. According to the 2001 U.S. Renal Data System (USRDS) Report, obstructive uropathy accounts for 9 percent of all end-stage renal disease in children.

Renal insufficiency in childhood results in many years of therapy. The USRDS reported in 2001 that the average cost of a year on kidney dialysis is $50,000. Numerous other persons with urethral valve obstruction suffer from mild to moderate renal insufficiency and have problems with urinary incontinence. Most require pharmacological and behavioral therapy.

Up to 5 percent of boys with posterior urethral valves will have voiding dysfunction that results in functional outlet obstruction. The consequences of this include recurrent UTI, vesicoureteral reflux (reflux of urine from the bladder into the ureters), and hydronephrosis (dilatation of one or both kidneys).

Severe functional bladder obstruction also occurs in children with spina bifida, who can develop both severe urinary incontinence and kidney changes. In addition, neurological disorders such as spinal cord injury, multiple sclerosis, and myelomeningocele often lead to voiding dysfunction characterized by functional bladder obstruction as a result of loss of coordination between the bladder and its outlet.

Groups at Risk

- *Aging men, who commonly develop benign prostatic hyperplasia (BPH)*

- *Children with developmental or congenital bladder obstruction (e.g., urethral valves)*

- *Adults and children with neurological disorders (e.g., spinal cord injury, multiple sclerosis, and myelomeningocele)*

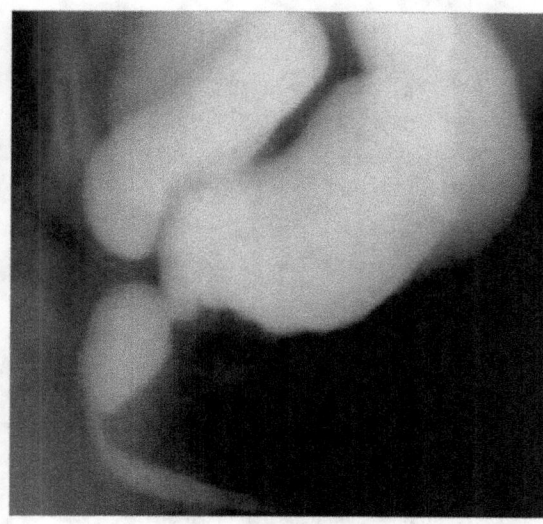

An x-ray of a boy with posterior urethral valves (PUV) and associated severe vesicoureteral reflux secondary to the PUV. Below the bladder (center), on the left, is the posterior urethra, which has become dilated as the result of obstruction by valves. Above the bladder and to the right and left are ureters, which are dilated from the abnormal reflux of urine on voiding.

Current Research

During the past decade, a substantial number of basic research grants from the National Institutes of Health (NIH) have been awarded for research that focused on bladder obstruction. This work has been highly productive, and knowledge gained from it has led to many more questions regarding the role of nerves, muscle, epithelium, matrix, and blood vessels in the development of lower urinary tract dysfunction and symptoms. Many of these issues are being investigated further in basic science research projects focused on these areas.

Funding for NIH Research

In fiscal year 2000, NIH-funded basic research on the effect of obstruction on bladder function was more limited than in previous years. A review of the portfolio identified a total of 10 individual NIH-funded grants. Although some overlap clearly exists between these grants in regard to research topics, the major topics included obstruction-induced changes in collagen expression, growth factors, contractile mechanisms, and metabolism. Only one grant focused on the effect of obstruction during development; the remainder dealt with obstruction in adults.

Major research topics that were not included in the portfolio included the effects of obstruction on the urothelium (epithelium), blood vessels, and nervous system, and the contribution of the nervous system to bladder symptoms induced by obstruction. In addition, the relevance of animal research to human research on bladder obstruction remains to be determined.

It is clear that only a small group of moderately experienced investigators is currently funded to study the effect of outlet obstruction on bladder function. The focus of these studies is relatively narrow in scope in comparison to the large number of important topics in this field. NIH currently funds two ongoing clinical studies of bladder obstruction. One is studying the effect of saw palmetto, an herbal product commonly used in alternative or complementary medicine to treat symptoms of BPH. The other is the multi-center study, Medical Therapy of Prostatic Symptoms (MTOPS), which is looking at the effect of the drug, Proscar, on prostatic obstruction, and comparing it with the effects of alpha-adrenergic blocking agents.

Recent Advances

Recent research has made several advances in the understanding of the mechanisms of obstruction and in the methods of treatment. These breakthroughs include improved understanding of the following:

- Alterations in the afferent (inflowing) and efferent (outflowing) nerves of the lower urinary tract after obstruction occurs

- Roles of physiological and biochemical factors related to, or dependent on, nutrition

- Roles of early response genes after outlet obstruction occurs

- Role of the ischemia-reperfusion cycle in bladder dysfunction after outlet obstruction occurs. (Obstruction causes a decrease in local blood flow [ischemia], and when blood flow is restored [reperfusion], tissue is often injured by the release of certain chemicals)

- Role of aging in the development of symptoms associated with bladder outlet obstruction, as is evident from the findings that elderly men and women have similar sensory symptoms

- Alternative therapies that may be effective in the treatment of obstructed bladder disorder

- Alterations in the extracellular matrix of the bladder that may be caused by outlet obstruction

- Treatment of BPH, which according to the results of the MTOPS study is effectively treated with two families of medications: one that decreases the size of the prostate and the other that alters bladder response to obstruction, either locally or centrally

Research Opportunities

Opportunities for research in bladder obstruction exist in the topic areas of genomics, cell regulation and signaling, technology, behavioral therapy, health services and outcomes, and groups with special needs.

Genomics

Identifying the genes in each bladder cell type that is modulated by obstruction is critical. Based on this information, it would be valuable to develop

- Gene arrays to allow for more detailed studies of cell and tissue changes that occur after obstruction develops

- Genetic therapies that respond to these genetic alterations

- Pharmacological interventions that target the protein consequences of these genetic changes

- Genetic markers associated with a high risk of bladder damage and failure from obstruction

- Genetic markers that predict reversibility and irreversibility of bladder decompensation

Cell Regulation and Signaling

Future research projects in cell regulation and signaling should

- Classify bladder obstruction based on the cellular and molecular changes that take place after obstruction

- Determine the time course of bladder obstruction based on the cellular and molecular changes that take place after obstruction

- Assess the differences in cell-cell interactions in the obstructed bladder compared with the normal bladder (compensated bladder compared with decompensated bladder)

- Target pharmacological therapy based on cell regulation and signaling

- Target pharmacological therapy based on the heterogeneity of bladder afferent nerves

Technology

Non-invasive technologies for the evaluation of bladder obstruction and its consequences are greatly needed. In particular, there is a need for non-invasive technologies for

- Diagnosis of obstruction (especially in children)

- Monitoring of the progression of obstruction from mild, compensated forms to severe, decompensated bladders

- Evaluation of the quality of bladder muscle, mucosa, and connective tissue

- Measurement of bladder oxygenation

- Functional metabolic imaging of the bladder

- Functional brain imaging to analyze changes in central neural pathways following bladder obstruction

Other technology needs include new and innovative techniques for

- Bladder replacement for treatment of end-stage bladder failure following obstruction

- Reduction of bladder outlet resistance

Behavioral Therapy

These investigations should include

- Trials of various forms of biofeedback on voiding dysfunction, particularly in children with urinary tract infections, reflux, and hydronephrosis

- Clinical studies of the effects of alternative therapies (e.g., acupuncture, herbal medications, phytotherapies, and magnet therapy) on bladder dysfunction related to obstruction

Health Services and Outcomes

Research studies of health services and outcomes should include

- Randomized prospective long-term studies comparing different methods of treating the lower urinary tract symptoms associated with obstruction

- Long-term outcome studies of the effect of urinary diversion and prophylactic therapy in children with bladder obstruction or neuropathic bladder

- Natural history of obstruction following anti-incontinence procedures

- Long-term outcome studies of pharmacologic therapy for prostatic obstruction

- Economic impact of sequential treatments of prostatic obstruction

- Natural history of sex differences in neonatal voiding

- Clinical trials based on cellular pathophysiology (e.g., free radical scavengers and growth factor agonists and antagonists)

Groups with Special Needs

Several groups have special needs that are critically important to study. Future research projects should focus on

- Differences in the response of the bladder to obstruction during growth and development

- Differences in the response of the bladder to obstruction during aging

Alterations of the bladder vasculature in response to obstruction

- Consequences of vascular disease on the response of the bladder to obstruction

- Reversibility of bladder dysfunction after release of obstruction

- Effects of male and female hormonal milieus on the effects of bladder obstruction

- Effects of the following on the response of the bladder to obstruction: systemic hormones (endocrine), hormones produced in and restricted to the local environment (paracrine), and cells that self-stimulate by producing a factor and also a receptor for that factor (autocrine)

Research Requirements

Manpower and infrastructure needs and the need for tissue banks must be addressed if research in bladder obstruction is to be successful.

Workforce

Incentives are critically needed for research in bladder obstruction. Few researchers have been interested in this area, and the number of grants is insufficient to encourage scientists to work in it. Training and development programs are needed as well as tuition and loan forgiveness. Incentives are needed to attract and retain residents, post-residents, and mid-level investigators.

Infrastructure

Because single institutions are unlikely to have the individual scientists needed to develop a critical mass, establishing multi-center research centers would allow interested researchers to collaborate productively.

Tissue and Specimen Banks

A critical deficiency in research today is the lack of human studies of bladder obstruction. A fundamental problem with carrying out meaningful research in human beings is the lack of suitably characterized tissue and specimen samples. One solution to this problem is tissue and specimen banking. Currently, three tissue repositories specifically study bladder tissue:

- The Interstitial Cystitis Multi-Center Study Group, which houses approximately 75 specimens and is funded by NIH

- The Cancer Center Tissue Core at the University of California, San Francisco, which is an inter-disciplinary group that consists of clinical and research scientists. Their tissue core collects fresh, frozen, and formalin-fixed, paraffin-embedded tissue from a variety of organs, including the bladder

- The Cell and Tissue Bank for Marker Studies of Diseases of the Bladder, Prostate, Kidney, Lung, and Breast, which is located in the Oklahoma City Veterans Medical Center. Bladder tissue and bladder washings are stored along with source character-ization and profiling

None of these tissue banks specifically collects tissue from obstructed human bladders or from suitable controls. The development of a tissue bank to study human bladder tissue is important. Urine and blood samples would also be useful because they may reflect bladder activity.

Other Needs

- Pharmaceutical and biotechnology interactions should be encouraged—especially for alternative therapies

- Public interest and educational efforts

- Ongoing review and advisory groups

Hayden Gantz

Posterior Urethral Valves, Obstructive Uropathy, Kidney Transplant

Hayden Gantz's mother, Carolyn, first noticed that his urine appeared cloudy when she began toilet training him at the age of 3. She took a urine sample to the laboratory at the children's hospital where she works as a nursing assistant, and had it examined. "It had all kinds of things in it that shouldn't be there," Gantz says. The presence of protein in urine makes it appear cloudy and is a sign of kidney disease.

Gantz immediately took her son to a physician who specializes in children's urologic problems. During the examination, the physician noticed "pus" in Hayden's diaper and admitted him to the hospital. Urinary tract infection, which is uncommon in boys at any age, is a sign of posterior urethral valves or PUV. Laboratory tests and radiography confirmed that Hayden had PUV, membranous folds in the posterior urethra that form during embryonic development and obstruct urine flow. In addition, one of Hayden's kidneys was so severely damaged from reflux of urine that it was not functioning. The other kidney was also damaged.

Posterior urethral valves are a life-threatening condition that occurs in approximately one in 8,000 newborn males. By the time many male infants with obstructive valves are born, they already have severe damage to their bladders and kidneys because as fetuses, they were unable to eliminate urine effectively. The high pressure produced by the blockage causes the bladder wall to thicken as the result of collagen deposition. Muscle tone declines and urine eventually refluxes back into the ureters and ultimately the kidneys, where the high pressure causes more damage and impairs kidney function. Once kidney damage occurs, secondary effects to other organ systems such as the lungs soon follow. Approximately one-third of children with posterior urethral valves progress to end-stage kidney disease and need kidney transplants.

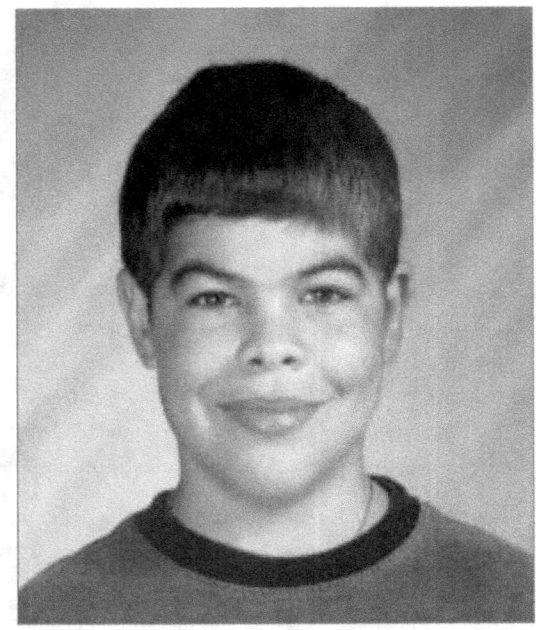

Today, diagnosis of urethral valves is often made by ultrasound during pregnancy. However, 12 years ago when Gantz was pregnant with Hayden, ultrasounds during pregnancy were rare, and even today, they are not routinely used. Also, according to some estimates, ultrasounds detect only 45 percent of children with valves. Children with mild cases can go undetected and are often not diagnosed until they are much older, when kidney damage has occurred.

Three days after being admitted to Children's Hospital, surgeons operated on Hayden to ablate the valves in his urethra and remove his non-functioning kidney and its ureter. They also tried to re-implant the other ureter into his bladder to correct the reflux and improve the function of the other kidney, but according to Gantz, they decided that this would not correct the problem.

"Hayden's bladder muscle was so stretched from the blockage that the bladder couldn't hold urine well," Gantz explains. "It leaked constantly." Instead, surgeons performed a ureterostomy, a surgical procedure that connects the ureter to a portion of the small intestine from which surgeons create an abdominal stoma or opening to the surface of the abdomen. Because the bladder is bypassed, urine flows through the stoma, located under the navel, into a bag that is glued to the skin.

Although the ureterostomy worked well during the seven years that Hayden grew from a toddler to a pre-teen, it also caused him many social problems that resulted in embarrassment and tears. Children who didn't understand Hayden's problem— and some who did—accused him of wetting his pants.

"Kids can be cruel," Ganz says. "His teachers worked with his classmates to explain some of the problems without going into too much detail, but many times Hayden came home in tears. At other times, he'd just shrug it off." Although Hayden wore baggy clothes to hide the pouch, it was more visible in summer because of lighter fabric. It also came off more frequently when he perspired or swam in the public pool. During one of these episodes, an inquisitive child asked Gantz if Hayden had been shot.

When Hayden was 10 years old, physicians who had been monitoring the deteriorating function of his remaining kidney decided that it was time to perform a transplant. Hayden was developing uremia, a build-up of urea and other nitrogenous wastes in the blood. But before the transplant could be done, Hayden had to undergo bladder dilatation in preparation for connecting his new kidney to the lower urinary tract. For three weeks, Gantz, who is a single parent, had to inject increasing amounts of sterile saline into her son's bladder up to 10 times a day, a process that was extremely painful in the beginning. Because Hayden's bladder was inactive for seven years, she explained, it could only hold 30 cc, a small amount. At the end of three weeks, his bladder was able to hold 500 cc, a normal amount.

"Pain is nothing new to Hayden," his mother sadly explains. "He's had a lot of painful things done to him over the years, but he's a real trooper."

In June 2001, after school had finished for the year, Hayden had a kidney transplant. The ureterostomy was repaired and the ureters from the new kidney were connected to his bladder. "The greatest words I've ever heard from my son were, 'Mom, I have to pee,'" says Gantz.

During the postoperative period, Hayden's new kidney functioned well, but his bladder and urethra were still a problem. His urethra had scar tissue where the valves were removed and this made urinating quite painful. In addition, the bladder muscle's tone was so poor it went into spasms, causing more pain, leakage, and frequent voiding. Hayden was reluctant to leave home for fear of being incontinent or having other children see him in pain, but bladder function eventually improved over the ensuing months and the urethral irritation subsided.

In the fall, Hayden had a temporary setback. He developed mononucleosis that required hospitalization because he is taking drugs to suppress his immune system. The drugs prevent rejection of his new kidney and he will be on them his entire life.

Today, "Hayden can do anything he wants except contact sports," his mother says. "In the beginning he had a few accidents and came home from school in tears, but now during the day, you would never know he has a bladder problem." Asleep, it's another problem. "He doesn't have a strong enough sensation during sleep to know that his bladder is full," Gantz explains. But she is used to this. "A lot of things have gotten wet over the years." It is another hurdle that she hopes Hayden will be able to surmount.

CHAPTER 8

INTERSTITIAL CYSTITIS

Common Clinical Conditions

DID YOU KNOW?

→ Although precise prevalence is unknown, interstitial cystitis (IC) has been estimated to affect 700,000 to 1 million people, 90 percent of whom are women.

→ The median age of onset is 40, but 25 percent of people who have IC are under 30 years old.

→ Some men diagnosed with non-bacterial prostatitis may in fact have IC.

→ People on kidney dialysis have been reported to have a better quality of life than people with IC.

→ Fifty percent of people with IC are unable to work full time.

→ IC is estimated to cost 1.7 billion dollars in medical expenses and lost wages annually.

Summary and Recommendations

Interstitial cystitis (IC) is a debilitating, chronic bladder syndrome that causes urinary urgency, frequency, and pain in the bladder and pelvic region. Some people with IC find that even a small amount of urine in the bladder causes discomfort, pressure, tenderness, or intense pain in that organ and in the surrounding pelvic region—symptoms that might resemble a urinary tract infection. However, analysis of a urine culture indicates no detectable infection, and symptoms of IC do not respond to anti-microbial therapies.

Although it affects mostly women, IC can occur in people of any age, sex, or race. The cause is unknown and the diagnosis is difficult. With neither a cure nor a consistently effective therapy available to treat it, IC has a negative impact on all aspects of a person's life. The pain of IC is often severe and can necessitate trips to the bathroom as often as every 15 minutes, both day and night. Severe symptoms leave many people home-bound and unable to socialize, sleep, work, or travel—deprivations that lead to depression and poor quality of life.

Although precise prevalence is unknown, as many as 700,000 to 1 million Americans may have IC, roughly equivalent to the number of people who have inflammatory bowel disease and Parkinson's disease. More people may have this condition, but have not yet been diagnosed.

After a comprehensive review of the current research on interstitial cystitis and the research opportunities available, the Bladder Research Progress Review Group (BRPRG) made the following high priority recommendations:

➡ **Investigate the cause and development of IC through studies that will also**

- Identify urinary, epithelial, inflammatory, vascular, and neurologic abnormalities

- Identify specific markers associated with pathogenesis, risk, disease activity, prognosis, response to therapy, and remission

- Classify subgroups of people based on abnormalities and markers

→ Conduct epidemiologic research, including population and case-control studies of incidence, prevalence, and natural history

→ Conduct clinical trials of novel therapies

→ Increase awareness of IC among the public and among health professionals

Background

Interstitial cystitis (IC) is one of the most challenging and frustrating problems facing people who have this disease, primary care providers, and urologists. At first glance, IC may be mistaken for a common, treatable bladder infection, thereby delaying accurate diagnosis. However, persistence of symptoms despite treatment with antibiotics and despite a urine culture that is negative for microorganisms may indicate IC rather than an uncomplicated urinary tract infection. People with IC face an illness that has potentially devastating physical, emotional, psychological, and socioeconomic consequences, an illness that is difficult to diagnose and has no uniformly effective treatment.

No blood or urine test is currently available to make diagnosis easy. Providers often consider IC only after ruling out other problems such as infections, bladder cancer, and bladder stones. Peering into the bladder using a cystoscope (a thin telescope), the urologist distends the bladder with fluid (hydrodistention) and sees an irritated, inflamed bladder, which also may be stiff and have scars, glomerulations, and Hunner's ulcers. Glomerulations are superficial areas of pinpoint bleeding caused by inflammation. Hunner's ulcers are stellate in form and are generally solitary and involve deeper layers of the bladder. Cystoscopy to visualize these changes is performed only when the person is under general or regional anesthesia.

The type and intensity of IC symptoms vary from person to person. Even in the same person, symptoms may range from annoying to incapacitating. People with IC feel an urgent or frequent need to urinate. Some find that even a small amount of urine in the bladder causes discomfort, pressure, tenderness, or intense pain, which can be felt not only in the bladder, but also in the surrounding pelvic region. Symptoms may change in intensity as the bladder fills with urine or as it empties, but frequency is not always related to bladder size; many people with severe frequency have normal bladder capacity. Sexual intercourse can also be painful for both men and women with IC, and intimacy is often impossible because of the severity of the pain. In women, symptoms of IC typically worsen around the time of menstruation. Severe symptoms leave many people homebound and unable to socialize, sleep, work, or travel—deprivations that lead to depression and a poor quality of life.

Etiology

Several theories about the cause of IC have arisen because of particular features of this condition. As a result, some experts have speculated that IC may actually include several sub-classes or separate diseases. One theory currently being investigated is that IC may be caused by a defect in the protective lining of the bladder, allowing substances in the urine to cause irritation. Another theory being investigated is that IC is an immunogenic or autoimmune condition. Neurogenic inflammation has also been posed as a contributing or causal factor in the development of IC.

Researchers are beginning to explore the possibility that heredity may play a part in IC. Recent genetic studies reveal an inherited susceptibility to IC among first-degree relatives and among some families with IC in multiple generations. To date, no gene has been implicated as a cause.

Research has recently shown that IC involves increased bladder permeability, mast cell activation, neurogenic inflammation, and various growth factors.

→ **Increased bladder permeability.** IC may be caused by a defect in the protective lining of the bladder, thereby allowing irritating substances in the urine to penetrate the bladder. This could result in symptoms of pain, urinary frequency, and urgency.

→ **Elevated number of mast cells.** Interstitial cystitis is associated with elevated mast cell counts in the bladder tissue. Mast cells produce many irritating substances, including histamine, eosinophilic chemotactic factor, and leukotrienes—substances that can contribute to inflammation and pain. Research evidence for mast cell involvement comes from a mouse model in which mast-cell-deficient mice exhibit a reduced sensitivity to the inflammatory mediator, lipopolysaccharide (LPS). Together, these findings suggest a pro-inflammatory model whereby substance P nerves of the bladder activate the mast cells, which in turn release potent inflammatory mediators and histamine, substances that can further antagonize nerves. A critical question in this model is, "What factor or factors initiate the loop?" This is an area of intense investigation.

→ **Neurogenic inflammation.** Pain is a common symptom of interstitial cystitis. It often persists even after the bladder has been removed, suggesting a strong central nervous system component. However, events originating in the nervous system that affect the bladder are also likely contributors to the pain of interstitial cystitis. Data point to a strong role for nerve pathways in interstitial cystitis pain, and continued efforts to identify the pain receptor pathways of the bladder are central to our understanding of this condition. Estrogen may enhance nerve growth factor expression in the bladder and contribute to inflammation of nerves, suggesting a basis for interstitial cystitis afflicting primarily females.

→ **Growth factors.** Heparin-binding epidermal-growth-factor-like growth factor (HB-EGF) has been found to be decreased in the urine of people with IC. This might inhibit the repair of the injured bladder lining, thereby contributing to the symptoms of IC. Also, research indicates that nerve growth factor (NGF) plays a role in IC.

Epidemiology

People of any age, race, or sex can have IC; however, approximately 90 percent of those with IC are women. Once thought to be a rare, post-menopausal disease, IC is now estimated to affect 700,000 to 1 million men, women, and children in the United States, a number that is roughly equivalent to the number of people who have inflammatory bowel disease and Parkinson's disease. Many more people are likely to have IC, but they have not yet been diagnosed or are misdiagnosed. On average, it takes five to seven years to obtain a diagnosis of IC.

According to data from the Nurses Health Studies I and II and from prior epidemiological studies, IC is more common among younger women. This debunks the myth that IC is exclusive to women who are post-menopausal. Symptoms of IC typically occur around age 40, but at least 25 percent of people with IC are younger than age 30. Studies also suggest that some men who have been diagnosed with non-bacterial prostatitis may actually have IC.

People with IC are also disproportionately diagnosed with diseases such as vulvodynia (burning and irritation in the vulva), allergies, irritable bowel syndrome, systemic lupus erythematosus (an autoimmune disease that results in episodes of inflammation of the joints, tendons, and other connective tissues and organs), inflammatory bowel disease (Crohn's disease and colitis), fibromyalgia (chronic widespread musculoskeletal pain and fatigue disorder of uncertain cause), and asthma. Some people have a genetic predisposition to these diseases, and this may be a factor for people with IC as well. The prevalence of IC among first-degree relatives is several times higher than the prevalence of IC in the general population. Preliminary data reveal that approximately 4 percent of people with IC have at least one family member with the condition. Additional studies into the genetics of IC, including linkage analysis, are now underway.

Cost and Impact

The economic impact of IC is significant. Symptoms are so severe that only about half of the estimated 700,000 to 1 million people with this disease are able to work full time. In 1988, that meant that IC accounted for an estimated $1.7 billion in medical expenses and lost wages, costs that would be significantly higher today considering rising costs and greater numbers of people with IC.

In addition to the financial considerations, the human toll can be devastating. According to one study, people with IC have a poorer quality of life than people who are on kidney dialysis because many become housebound, unemployed, and unable to enjoy hobbies, a restaurant meal, a movie, travel, physical intimacy, or other simple pleasures that contribute to living a good life.

Current Research

The IC research program began at the National Institute of Diabetes and Digestive and Kidney Diseases (NIDDK) in 1987 with two clinical grants and five basic research grants totaling $1.1 million. Thanks to strong congressional support, the program has grown dramatically and in fiscal year 2000 included a record 46 grants totaling $11.2 million, including basic research on underlying bladder dysfunction and clinical research. The investment has led to a better understanding of the problem. NIDDK's IC database was the first systematic, multi-center, observational, longitudinal effort to collect demographic, dietary, diagnostic, symptom, treatment, and other information from a large number of people with the condition. The database also laid the groundwork for NIDDK's IC Clinical Trials Group (ICCTG), a consortium to test potential treatments.

The ICCTG is also gathering information that researchers hope will provide better methods for diagnosing IC. The October 2000 meeting, "Interstitial Cystitis and Bladder Research: Progress and Future Directions," encouraged scientists to share research ideas and results. The Interstitial Cystitis Association, an advocacy group for people with IC, and the NIDDK both co-sponsored the meeting.

Men with non-bacterial prostatitis (NBP) may also benefit from clinical research on IC, since non-bacterial prostatitis is a similar condition. Some experts suggest that NBP may be the male equivalent of IC. However, preliminary data reveal that antiproliferative factor (APF), a marker unique to people with IC, is rarely found in men with benign prostatic hyperplasia (BPH), a condition that often causes inflammation of the prostate. Some of the same researchers are studying both conditions, increasing opportunities for the cross-fertilization of ideas relevant to both conditions.

NIDDK hopes to extend the breadth and depth of the IC research program to understudied areas of high priority by supporting projects that will increase understanding of the fundamental needs for normal bladder function and the errors that lead to dysfunction by attracting talented investigators from other fields and by collecting and analyzing more and better data on IC.

Based on expert recommendations, NIDDK is planning a two-pronged approach to epidemiological studies. In the first approach, the *Urology in America Database* will be mined for physician and hospital costs and the frequency of bladder and other urinary tract disorders. In the second approach, reliable data will be obtained to more accurately estimate the number of men and women who have chronic painful bladder syndromes such as IC and to identify the degree of disability caused by these conditions. This latter initiative began in FY 2001, with projects funded under the request for application (RFA), "Epidemiology of Chronic Pelvic Pain of the Bladder and Interstitial Cystitis."

Highlights of Currently Funded NIDDK Research

NIDDK's Interstitial Cystitis Clinical Trials Group (ICCTG), a consortium of nine clinical centers across the country, is evaluating the safety and efficacy of various treatments for IC. Currently, ICCTG is studying an innovative intravesical treatment involving a bacterium known as bacillus Calmette-Guerin (BCG). BCG is thought to work by stimulating the immune system.

The NIDDK has also investigated or continues to investigate the following areas:

- Role of nitric oxide

- Sensory and sympathetic nervous system effects

- Afferent mechanisms underlying bladder pain

- Urine and bladder diagnostic markers

- Pain sensitivity and menstrual cycle effects

- Urine anti-proliferative peptides

- Chronic pelvic pain of the bladder and IC (epidemiology RFA to be funded)

- Neurogenic inflammation

- Stress-induced neuroinflammatory changes

- Quantitative study of urinary bladder sensory processing

- Immune mediators

- Nitric oxide transduction mechanisms in UTI and IC

- Studies of pain in people with IC

- Afferent plasticity underlying urethral and pelvic pain

Two specific areas of investigation include diagnostic markers and tests and new treatments.

Diagnostic Markers and Tests

Efforts are underway to find less painful, less invasive, and more accurate diagnostic tests for IC. At present, clinical findings of urinary urgency, frequency, and pain in the absence of other urologic conditions, along with the presence of glomerulations or Hunner's ulcers on cystoscopy, are considered to be the gold standard for the diagnosis of IC. However, urinary markers hold great promise for potential development into a clinical test and may provide clues into the cause and treatment of IC. Markers are unique factors found in a particular disorder that can be recognized and identified. Conclusive diagnosis of IC using a marker would enhance both epidemiologic and biologic studies of its pathophysiology.

Researchers have identified the following factors that may explain the changes in the bladder that occur with IC:

- Heparin-binding-epidermal-growth-factor-like growth factor (HB-EGF)—HB-EGF is important for epithelial cell proliferation and wound healing. In one study, urine and blood samples were obtained from three groups: people who were asymptomatic, people with IC, and people with urologic conditions other than IC, including those with urinary tract infections. HB-EGF levels were significantly decreased only in the urine and serum of people with IC. These findings suggest that the lack of HB-EGF may be responsible for the bladder's inability to repair damaged epithelium. The presence of decreased levels of HB-EGF in the serum of people with IC suggests that IC may be a systemic disease.

- Anti-proliferative factor (APF) — Anti-proliferative factor is found only in the urine of people with IC. This protein inhibits HB-EGF production and may prevent the growth of new, healthy bladder epithelium.

Both HB-EGF and APF were confirmed as markers for IC in a recent blinded study. These research findings could lead to a diagnostic test and the identification of agents to suppress production of APF, block its actions, or enhance production of the epithelial growth factor, allowing the growth of healthy bladder cells lining the bladder.

Additional urinary markers that might be useful as diagnostic markers or objective measures of treatment response were recently confirmed in another study. Interleukin-6 (IL-6) was found to be increased in some people with IC and may be produced by inflammatory or bladder epithelial cells. Studies have also shown that cyclic GMP (guanosine monophosphate), a factor necessary for the synthesis of DNA and RNA, is also decreased in people with IC. Epidermal growth factor (EGF) has been confirmed to be significantly elevated in the urine of people with IC, as well.

A lactulose-rhamnose test, similar to the test used to diagnose gastrointestinal permeability, is also being investigated. This test for bladder permeability involves instilling a sugar solution into the bladder and subsequently checking for levels of this sugar molecule in the serum. Far less invasive to the patient when compared to cystoscopy and hydrodistention under general anesthesia, this new permeability test may distinguish intact bladders from permeable bladders.

These new tests and markers currently under investigation will undoubtedly help to make the diagnosis and treatment of IC more accurate and less painful in the future.

Potential Treatments

The NIDDK's ICCTG is evaluating the safety and efficacy of potential treatments. The first trial by this consortium tested oral medications, pentosan polysulfate sodium (Elmiron®) and hydroxyzine hydrochloride (Atarax®). Earlier studies suggested that each drug targets different aspects of IC. Elmiron® the first oral medication approved for IC, reinforces the bladder lining, which usually acts as a barrier to the toxicity of urine, whereas Atarax® an antihistamine, reduces the activity of mast cells, which may cause bladder inflammation and pain. The two drugs may also work synergistically, leading to quicker, more potent symptom relief.

The second ICCTG clinical trial is testing whether the bacterium, bacillus Calmette-Guérin (BCG), will relieve the pelvic pain and frequent urination that are hallmarks of IC. Earlier studies in people with IC suggest that BCG stimulates a protective immune response (the production of type 1 T helper cells) and downplays a harmful immune response (production of type 2 T helper cells) in the bladders of people with IC. Results of both clinical trials will be announced on NIDDK's website (www.niddk.nih.gov) when they become available.

Other new treatments being tested by pharmaceutical companies include Resiniferatoxin, (RTX), sacral nerve stimulation devices, hyaluronic acid (Cystistat.), and SI-7201 (sodium hyaluronate).

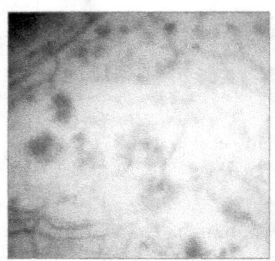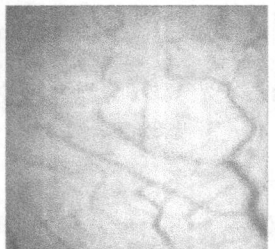

Cystoscopic images showing (left) glomerulations–tiny hemorrhages that are a telltale sign of interstitial cystitis–and (right) a healthy bladder. (*Photo Credit: Healthcommunities.com, Inc., interstitial cystitis on urologychannel.® http://www.urologychannel.com/interstitialcystitis. Copyright® 2002, Healthcommunities.com, Inc.*)

Critical Research Areas

The usefulness of the NIDDK criteria for IC research needs to be re-established, and a consensus conference on the definition and diagnosis of IC is urgently needed to assist the practicing clinician as well as to establish guidelines for future research.

The following areas have been defined by the BRPRG as being critical to IC research, and resources should be directed towards them:

- Etiology and pathogenesis
- Epidemiology
- Disease markers
- Molecular biology
- Genetics
- Neurological aspects

Etiology and Pathogenesis

Arguably, this is the most important research area in IC. Well-designed studies of clinical patients and material should be directed at understanding the primary defect and the subsequent disease development sequence (pathogenesis) in IC. These studies conceivably could include one or more of the following areas: urine, epithelium, blood vessels, inflammatory response, neurologic activity, or pelvic floor dysfunction.

Specific urinary markers that may indicate a mechanism of pathogenesis should also be studied further. One such marker, anti-proliferative factor (APF), has been shown to alter the production of at least three growth factors and one growth-factor-binding protein by bladder epithelial cells *in vitro*. Additional studies on the acute and chronic effects of APF on epithelial function and mechanisms of growth factor regulation (e.g., release of signaling molecules and formation of tight junctions) are warranted. Studies on the role of other markers in IC (including interleukin-6 and cyclic GMP) should also be pursued.

Collaborative research on the cause and pathogenesis of IC and associated disorders—vulvodynia, allergies, irritable bowel syndrome, lupus, fibromyalgia, asthma, Crohn's disease, colitis, and Sjögren's Syndrome—should be studied .

Epidemiology

Population-based studies would give the most accurate data on incidence, prevalence, and potential risk factors and identify a cohort of incident cases, which is critical to understanding the etiology and natural history of this disease.

The identification of IC cases compared to appropriately matched controls is the most cost-effective method of identifying risk factors, demographic features, familial aggregation, and non-urinary clinical syndromes associated with IC. Enrichment of such case control studies by new onset cases will allow important investigations of recent antecedent events and of early urine, serum, and histopathologic factors that might provide clues to the development of the disease.

Large cohorts of persons who do not have IC, along with baseline data and specimens, would allow identification of incident cases with not only the advantages attendant to study of new onset cases as above, but also the availability of pre-IC urine and blood specimens allowing a search for causative factors. Identification of new cases and banking of such specimens could be incorporated into ongoing large cohort studies such as the Nurses' Health Study I and II.

Finally, longitudinal studies of people with IC would be appropriate to define natural history, including prognosis, prognostic factors, and incidence of complications and aggravating events. Identifying cohorts of persons with IC that were established sometime in the past (such as those in the IC Database or those who participated in earlier therapeutic trials) could minimize the expense of this type of study. These people could be re-enrolled with appropriate collection of data and then prospectively followed.

Disease Markers

The identification of a diagnostic marker that has excellent sensitivity, specificity, positive predictive value, and negative predictive value and that does not require an expensive or invasive technique (e.g., cystoscopy with hydrodistention under general anesthesia) is critical. A number of markers have been reported by numerous investigators and are being compared in the same patient group. The most promising diagnostic markers identified in recent blinded studies include anti-proliferative factor (APF), heparin-binding-epidermal-growth factor-like growth factor (HB-EGF), and epidermal growth factor (EGF). The markers should be studied further, and one or two markers should be included in all subsequent clinical and epidemiologic studies to confirm diagnostic capability and to determine usefulness in predicting prognosis or in monitoring natural history or therapy.

At this point in time, IC is a field driven almost exclusively by clinical observations. It would seem that this field is ideally suited to translational research; however, given the lack of knowledge of the cause and natural history of IC, a reverse approach would be appropriate. This approach would look at the clinical course of persons with IC and identify responders to treatment, non-responders, and those in spontaneous remission. Serum, urine, and tissue specimens could be collected from people with IC and from control groups to identify abnormal gene expression patterns in people with IC using proteomics and cDNA micro-array technology. This approach might identify additional disease markers and lead to greater understanding of the mechanisms involved in the development of IC.

Molecular Biology

An understanding of the cellular gene expression of bladder tissues that differ between persons with IC and persons who are "normal" could lead to an understanding of the pathogenesis of IC. Development of certain tools, including microarrays for human bladder epithelial cells would be useful for these studies. It is possible that different molecular targets will be identified in different subgroups of people with IC. Identifying subgroups could lead to targeted treatments.

The application of new technology developed in the field of cancer could dramatically advance current research in IC. These advances allow the isolation of pure populations of individual cell types in sufficient cell numbers to analyze their gene and protein expression. Laser capture microdissection (LCM) will allow the isolation of pure populations of lymphoid cells and epithelium from people with IC and from normal controls for gene and protein profiling. For example, proteomics technologies such as mass-spectroscopy can isolate, characterize, and define proteins in the urine. Using these methodologies, new tests to diagnose and monitor IC could be developed, and persons with IC could be classified into subgroups based on protein expression. These technologies are valuable because they do not involve an invasive procedure and could also be used after treatment to define changes at the protein level.

Genetics

Preliminary published reports indicate a higher-than-expected prevalence of IC among first-degree relatives of index IC cases, concordance among monozygotic (identical) twins for IC, and several families with IC in multiple generations. These findings are consistent with an inherited susceptibility to IC. Linkage analysis and positional cloning can be used to identify location of susceptibility gene(s) to IC. The rapid progress being made in sequencing the human genome will facilitate identification of such genes.

Neurologic Aspects

The nerve-cell-like properties of epithelial cells should be examined to identify how these properties are changed in people with IC. These properties include the release of transmitters (i.e., nitric oxide and adenosine triphosphate [ATP]), the expression of transmitter receptors (i.e., cholinergic, adrenergic, serotonergic, and capsaicin receptors), response to transmitters, communication with afferent (inflowing) nerve cells, communication with efferent (outflowing) nerve cells, and intracellular signaling mechanisms that mediate transmitter actions.

The properties of bladder afferent nerve cells should be studied in more detail, particularly those involved in triggering painful sensations. Topics for research should include

- Mechanisms that underlie acute and chronic sensitization of afferent receptors

- Identification of molecular targets for the pharmacologic modulation of afferent excitability

- Changes in the expression of ion channels and receptors in chronic pathological conditions

- Cross-talk between afferent and efferent nerves or between epithelial cells and afferent nerves

- Mechanisms involved in the central processing of afferent input from the bladder, including neurotransmitters, plasticity induced by chronic pathological conditions, and targets for pharmacotherapy of bladder pain

Early Diagnosis and Treatment

Early diagnosis could be helpful in avoiding the dramatic physical, psychological, and socioeconomic impact of IC and in facilitating a higher likelihood of response to treatment. Physician education and public awareness are imperative. Treatment of this devastating condition has not been fundamentally improved over many years, and investigators cannot wait for the aforementioned goals to come to fruition before focusing on new treatment modalities for this group of people. Good clinical trials are imperative. Clinical studies should be combined with basic science (i.e., markers and genomic and proteomic studies). Promising therapies should be studied in a controlled multi-center manner as is currently being done by the NIDDK IC Clinical Trials Group.

Additional Opportunities for Research

Research areas such as animal models, the pathophysiology of symptom production, the IC Database, and normal bladder structure and function would also be extremely valuable.

Animal Models

Progress in understanding the pathogenesis of IC comes with the development of faithful model systems. Currently, few model systems exist for the study of IC. A feline model exhibits many similarities to human IC, but the prevalence of IC among cats is not high. In addition, this model is not easily amenable to experimental manipulation or genetic analysis. An acute rat model of neurogenic cystitis based on infection with neurotrophic pseudo-rabies virus (PRV) shows promise for experimental manipulation, but the systemic effects of PRV limit the use of this model for characterizing chronic aspects of IC.

Valid *in vitro* IC models that mimic the important cell-to-cell interactions in the bladder are also needed because such a system could be easily manipulated. Thus, the development of better *in vitro* and *in vivo* models for the study of interstitial cystitis is clearly needed.

Two types of animal experiments would be useful in understanding IC:

- Animal experiments using agents that result in urgency, frequency, and pain in the animal model

- Subsequent studies to look at the mechanism of this effect, to identify markers and molecular targets associated with the above symptoms, and to investigate possible therapeutic interventions

Studies should be performed to test cause-and-effect hypotheses through the use of precise physiologic defects engineered by drugs or genetic knockout animals. Additional studies on Feline Urologic Syndrome, a naturally occurring bladder disorder in cats that mimics certain features of human IC, are also warranted.

Pathophysiology of Symptom Production

Whether an etiology for IC is known or not, an understanding of the means by which the symptoms of IC are produced may lead to new and effective interventions.

Interstitial Cystitis Data Base (ICDB)

Much data have been collected by the Interstitial Cystitis Data Base (ICDB) and should be analyzed to increase our understanding of IC. For instance, the database could provide answers to the following questions:

- What pathologic features are associated with what symptoms of IC?

- Is hydrodistention necessary for diagnosis in people with appropriate symptoms, negative urine culture, and negative pre-hydrodistention cystoscopy?

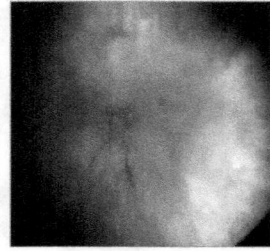 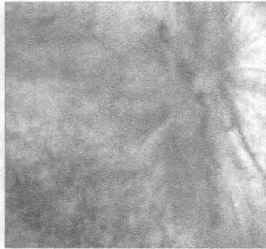

Hunner's ulcers in a patient with interstitial cystitis. The image on the right clearly shows the common stellate pattern of the ulcer. As is typical, the center of the lesion has a large amount of granulation tissue present, probably as a result of small tears and bleeding that may occur with bladder filling. *(Photo Credit: Dr. Robert Moldwin, Albert Einstein College of Medicine, Bronx, NY)*

- Is a biopsy necessary for diagnosis?

- Are urodynamics studies necessary for diagnosis?

Answers to these and certain other questions may be within the ICDB. Newer additional data should be included in order to gain a better understanding of the pathophysiology of IC. This data would provide a newer perspective, since the definition, diagnosis, and treatment of IC have substantially evolved since 1991, when the ICDB was started.

Normal Bladder Structure and Function

Not enough is known about the normal bladder. Studies including, but not limited to, epithelial differentiation, proliferation and migration, hormonal response and receptors, and epithelial antigen presentation would ultimately have effects upon our understanding of IC. Studies to identify specific physiologic interactions between and among different bladder wall components would be useful. Finally, development of *in vitro*, multi-layered, differentiated human bladder epithelium would allow studies to better determine regulation of normal bladder epithelial cell proliferation and differentiation.

Outside Sources for Research

The Interstitial Cystitis Association's Pilot Research Program and the Fishbein Family Interstitial Cystitis Research Foundation both provide funding for pilot projects specifically on interstitial cystitis. These pilot research grants have enabled researchers to study new ideas and obtain preliminary data. They have also attracted new researchers to this growing field. Many recipients of these pilot grants have gone on to receive NIH funding. Much of the pilot research funded over the past decade has resulted in important advances in the field of IC research, including urinary markers and the genetics of IC.

Research Requirements and Impediments

Requirements

→ **Workforce.** Encouraging career development in urology, urogynecology, and urologic research is essential. The growing fields of women's urology and urogynecology appear to be merging. This provides potential opportunities for an academic career for residents and fellows, but only if funding is provided to them early on. For example, the American Foundation for Urologic Disease (AFUD) administers a successful research scholars program that fosters careers in urologic research by providing young researchers with grant opportunities during their urologic fellowships. Additional programs are imperative to attract bright talented researchers, especially in today's challenging medical climate, where the costs of medical education are high.

→ **Tissue banks.** A large quantity of material—serum, urine, and biopsy specimens—is available from the NIDDK IC Data Base (ICBD). Urine specimens from the current NIDDK IC Clinical Trials Group are also being banked.

→ **Pharmaceutical and biotechnology efforts.** The pharmaceutical industry has shown significant interest in developing therapies for urinary urgency and frequency and for evaluating these therapies once FDA approval has been obtained. These therapies include bacillus Calmette-Guerin (BCG), resiniferatoxin (RTX,), hyaluronic acid (Cystistat,), sodium hyaluronate (SI-7201), and sacral nerve stimulation devices.

Impediments

- Delay in diagnosis and treatment
- Lack of a clinically available specific test for IC
- Lack of awareness within the medical community
- Lack of public awareness
- Lack of epidemiologic data
- Poor understanding of etiology and pathogenesis
- Lack of adequate treatments and pain management

Kara Fishbein Goldman

Interstitial Cystitis

In 1994, when she was barely 20 years old and a student at the University of Pennsylvania, Kara Fishbein Goldman was diagnosed with interstitial cystitis or IC. She did not have too many symptoms of IC at that time, she says, but she had vulvodynia, chronic pain in the vulva, a symptom often associated with IC.

While Goldman was under anesthesia for treatment of the vulvodynia, her doctor dilated the bladder with sterile saline solution and used a cystoscope to visualize the bladder wall. He found areas of inflammation and pinpoint bleeding called glomerulations, which are characteristic of IC. Eventually, Goldman developed other symptoms of the disease—urinary frequency, urgency, and a burning sensation in the bladder—symptoms that she has experienced constantly for the past eight years.

Goldman describes her pain as feeling as though she has a bad bladder infection—a burning type pain that gets worse as her bladder becomes full—but "antibiotics don't cure it and other medications provide little relief," she says. "I feel like I have to [urinate] all the time, and it gets worse when the bladder is full. The pain is constant, but the severity varies."

Symptoms of IC vary from patient to patient, but they generally cluster around an urgent need to urinate; frequent urination both day and night; reduced bladder capacity; and feelings of pressure, tenderness, and pain around the bladder, pelvis, and genital area that may increase as the bladder fills.

"With IC, everybody is different. The pain presents in different ways in different people," Goldman explains. "Some have sharp pain, some have a burning sensation all the time where the inside of your body feels like it's on fire." She believes IC is more like a syndrome, a collection of symptoms. "Some people have some symptoms from the syndrome. Some people have other symptoms from the syndrome." In fact, Goldman's

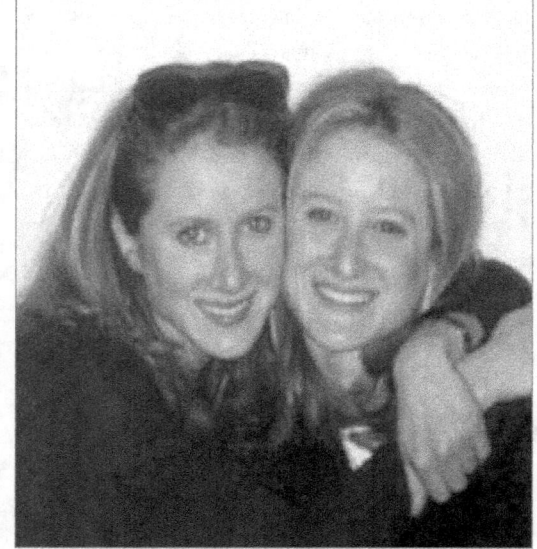

From left, Kara and Beth Fishbein

identical twin, Beth Fishbein, who developed IC a year after she did, has had milder symptoms. Currently in medical school, Fishbein is stabilized on a low dose of medication.

In some ways, Goldman and her sister were lucky. Their IC was diagnosed in the early stages, obviating the need to search for a diagnosis, a frustrating journey most people with IC are forced to undertake because many physicians are unfamiliar with the condition or because symptoms are often confused with other illnesses such as urinary tract infections. Even after IC has been diagnosed, many patients still have to search for new or different treatments that may help with their particular symptoms.

In the year after her diagnosis, Goldman instilled a weekly "cocktail" of medications prescribed by her physician into her bladder through self-catheterization. The bladder instillation included a local anesthetic, an antibiotic, and a steroid to reduce inflammation. This regimen kept her symptoms under control for about a year, but then the "cocktail" ceased to be effective, Goldman says, so she stopped it. Her pain gradually got worse, and became difficult to manage in the year before her wedding. She tried numerous oral medications, including tricyclic antidepressants, drugs that relax the bladder muscle, block pain, and have some effect on the body's allergic response, which appears to be involved in IC. Other drugs prescribed for her condition include a drug to relieve nerve pain; a drug that appears to augment the bladder lining; several pain medications; and drugs to relieve the bladder spasms that often accompany and worsen urinary urgency, frequency, and pain. All of the medications helped for only a little while, Goldman says, and a neurostimulation device implanted in the epidural space of her sacrum did not provide any relief.

Interstitial cystitis has no cure and no universal treatment; therefore, physicians must try several treatments to relieve symptoms. People with IC have responded to various therapies, but even so, a particular treatment may work only temporarily. Flare-ups and remissions also occur.

"The [pain medicine] doesn't ever make my pain go away," she says, "It just makes me tired and sleepy and less aware of myself." This creates a dilemma. She either works in pain or takes off and sleeps. During the workday, Goldman forgoes the pain medicine, but when the pain is severe, she takes off from work, takes the medicine, and sleeps. She says she's lucky because some people wake up from the pain; she does not.

"There's nothing much I can do to make myself feel better," she says. "I'm either working or sleeping. I don't want to sleep the rest of my life."

Goldman has tried to explain her illness to her students, co-workers, and friends to help them understand why she cannot function as well as she would like. She has had varying degrees of success. "People don't understand chronic pain," she says. "I look absolutely fine, and people can't see that I'm in pain. I'm not limping and I don't look particularly bad." Last October and this spring, Goldman's pain was so severe she had to take quite a number of days off from her teaching job. "This year was really bad. I missed a lot of days of school, and I'm taking a leave of absence [next school term]. This illness has affected my life in a big way," Goldman says, adding that she and her husband, Steve, had hoped to have children by now, but can't because of all the medications she's on.

Goldman says she feels fortunate to have an extremely supportive and caring spouse and parents, who have been very helpful in her often frustrating search for therapy that will ease her symptoms. In 1997, after realizing that scientists knew very little about IC, Goldman's parents, Bob and Laurie Fishbein, established the Fishbein Family Interstitial Cystitis Research Foundation, which endows pilot studies of IC. Goldman also acknowledges great support from the Interstitial Cystitis Association, which has provided her with information about IC and treatment options and has put her in touch with other people with IC.

So far, Goldman's search for effective treatment and pain relief has taken her to six gynecologists, three urologists, and two pain specialists in two states. She hopes that her yearlong leave from teaching will lead to better health and perhaps to the fulfillment of a long-delayed goal. "I want to be free to go wherever I need to go in the country to see consultants," she says. "I'll take it easy and try to feel better. Maybe if I can get off the drugs, I'll try to get pregnant…. I'll revise as I go. I'll keep trying different things."

CHAPTER 9

URINARY TRACT INFECTIONS

Common Clinical Conditions

DID YOU KNOW?

→ Urinary tract infections (UTIs) are responsible for an estimated seven million visits to doctors' offices.

→ UTIs cause approximately one million visits to emergency departments each year.

→ Adult women have about a 50 percent lifetime risk of developing a UTI.

→ Globally, direct costs of UTI are estimated to be $6 billion annually.

→ Catheter-related UTIs account for 40 percent of all hospital-acquired infections.

Summary and Recommendations

Urinary tract infections (UTIs) are common problems in men and women of all ages. However, certain groups have a greater risk of developing them. In particular, females are far more likely than males to develop a UTI, except in the first few months of life. In the United States, an estimated seven million cases of uncomplicated UTI occur annually in women, and approximately a third of the women who have an initial infection will develop a recurrence. Although few studies have been done on post-menopausal women, about 10 percent to 15 percent of this population experience recurrent UTIs.

Other groups at increased risk for developing UTIs are infants; pregnant women; the elderly; and persons with spinal cord injuries, catheters, diabetes, multiple sclerosis, and urologic abnormalities. UTIs in children cause significant morbidity and may lead to end-stage kidney disease. UTIs also cause significant morbidity and mortality in elderly men and women.

Better studies of the incidence of UTIs research are needed. It has been estimated that fewer than 70 investigators work in UTI research throughout the world and that only $20 million is spent on UTI research per annum. Currently, determinations of incidence are largely based on analyses of poorly documented, small, non-representative databases. Prospective, population-based studies are also critically needed. The Bladder Research Progress Review Group (BRPRG) has conducted a comprehensive study of current research on urinary tract infections and inflammation and recommends that the research community do the following:

→ **Increase basic and clinical research to study the processes of infection of the bladder.** Areas of interest and goals for future research include

- Bacterial pathogenesis

- Host tissue and innate immune responses

- Host adaptive immune responses

- Host susceptibility to infection and inflammation

- Comprehensive epidemiological studies of UTI

- Prevention and treatment of UTIs in normal and special hosts

➡ **Create new regional centers equipped with advanced technologies for genetic, proteomic, and functional bacterial and cellular arrays.** The regional centers should also be equipped with related technologies necessary for contemporary research in infection of the bladder. Ongoing support for the operation of these centers and technologies should also be provided.

Background

Urinary tract infections (UTIs) are frequently encountered in clinical practice. Classifications of the various clinical forms of UTI have been devised to account for differences in pathogenic mechanisms, sites of disease, and other host factors such as comorbidities (concomitant but unrelated disease processes). For example, UTIs are often classified as either uncomplicated or complicated.

- Uncomplicated UTIs occur in persons, primarily women, whose urinary tracts are normal in anatomy and function.

- Complicated UTIs occur in children and in persons who have underlying medical conditions that render infections more difficult to diagnose and treat. People with complicated UTIs require greater medical vigilance both before and after treatment. Serious forms of UTI require hospitalization or extended hospital stays that are very costly.

Urinary tract infections in adults may also be classified into other clinical categories, including acute or recurrent UTI, acute kidney infection, catheter-associated UTI, and urosepsis, invasion of surrounding tissues and the blood stream by pathogens that originally infected the urinary tract.

Incidence and Prevalence

Urinary tract infections are not reportable diseases in the United States; therefore, accurate incidence data are lacking. Estimates often differ depending on the diagnostic criteria (e.g., clinical presentation, urinalysis, and culture) and the situation in which the criteria were used (e.g., office visit, hospital discharge, self-report or physician diagnosis, and population screening). According to the most recent epidemiologic data from the 1997 National Ambulatory Medical Care Survey and the 1997 National Hospital Ambulatory Medical Care Survey, UTIs are the reason for nearly seven million office visits each year and another one million emergency department visits, resulting in approximately 100,000 hospitalizations.

UTIs are more common in females than in males, except in the first few months of life. Adult women have about a 50 percent lifetime risk of developing a UTI. One study of first-time, symptomatic UTI in children younger than age six estimated that girls have three times the risk of boys for developing a UTI. Symptomatic UTI is also common among young, sexually active, adult women, ages 18 to 29.

The overall prevalence of bacteria in the urine (bacteriuria) that do not produce symptoms (asymptomatic bacteriuria) has been estimated at 5 percent in young, ambulatory women, and prevalence generally increases with age in both women and men. Asymptomatic bacteriuria is particularly serious in pregnant women, although only a small percentage of them are diagnosed with it. This condition is associated with adverse effects on the newborn and an abnormal course of pregnancy. The incidence increases with age, the number of times a woman has given birth (parity), diabetes, and history of UTI.

Both asymptomatic bacteriuria and symptomatic UTI have been reported to be more prevalent among women with diabetes than among men with the disease. Women also reportedly have three times as many hospitalizations for an acute kidney infection than their male counterparts.

> **Conditions that Complicate a UTI**
>
> - *Extremes of age (children or elderly adults)*
>
> - *Anatomic abnormalities of the urinary tract*
>
> - *Metabolic and hormonal abnormalities (e.g., diabetes)*
>
> - *Impaired host defenses*
>
> - *Medical conditions affecting urinary tract function*
>
> - *Catheterization*

Among people older than age 70 who are living independently, the incidence of asymptomatic bacteriuria has been estimated to be three times greater for women (16 percent to 18 percent) than for men (6 percent). However, studies that categorize prostatitis (inflammation or infection of the prostate gland) with UTI have found nearly comparable rates among older men and women.

In addition to pregnant women, infants, and the elderly, other populations are also at increased risk; these include persons with spinal cord injuries, catheters, diabetes, urologic abnormalities, and multiple sclerosis (MS). People with MS appear to be at significant increased risk of UTI. In one study of urinary tract dysfunction in people with MS, nearly 90 percent had urinary tract infections, with bacteriuria affecting up to 74 percent. A UTI frequently precedes relapse of MS symptoms, and recurrent UTIs have been associated with acute exacerbation and neurologic progression of MS.

HIV status appears to be another risk factor for UTI. Studies have reported that the incidence of UTI among women and men who are HIV positive is greater than the incidence among women and men who are HIV negative.

In addition, UTIs currently account for more than a third of the two million infections that occur in hospitals each year. Most of these UTIs are secondary to an indwelling urethral catheter. Catheter-related UTI has been estimated to be responsible for 40 percent of all institution-related infections. Although a decrease has occurred in catheter-related UTI rates among patients in intensive care units during the past decade, the rates remain high.

Cost and Impact

Even if it is uncomplicated, a urinary tract infection reportedly causes adults six days of frequent and painful urinations, including two days of reduced activity and at least one day of missed work. When a UTI occurs in a young child, these costs frequently involve hospitalization and loss of work for the parents. The financial and medical implications are enormous, in part because UTI is such a common disease. Direct costs of UTI include medical charges for doctor visits and drugs and non-medical costs associated with travel, sick days, and morbidity. Indirect costs associated with lost output must also be considered.

The total annual cost of UTIs in the United States has been estimated to be greater than $1 billion, and this estimate does not include hospital costs. Annual direct costs of UTI in women have been reported to be $659 million and indirect costs, $936 million. Moreover, annual costs of hospital-related UTIs have been estimated to range between $424 million and $451 million. Catheter-related UTIs, which are responsible for well over a third of all hospital-related infections, significantly increase the cost and impact of UTIs.

Groups at Risk

Infants and Children

Approximately 18 percent of infants who develop a UTI during their first year of life experience a recurrence during the subsequent months. Recurrent urinary tract infections in infants and children are associated with significantly greater morbidity, including impaired kidney function, end-stage kidney disease, and possible complications of pregnancy.

> ### Who's at Risk for UTI?
>
> - *Infants and children*
>
> - *People with catheters, spina bifida, spinal cord injuries, and diabetes*
>
> - *Pregnant women*
>
> - *The elderly*
>
> - *People with renal transplants*
>
> - *People in certain racial and ethnic groups*

Approximately 3 percent of prepubertal girls and 1 percent of prepubertal boys are diagnosed annually with UTIs. The clinical course and sequelae of UTI in children is different from that of adults. Guidelines developed by the American Academy of Pediatrics recommend that children ages two months to two years who have an unexplained fever should be evaluated for a UTI because of its serious potential consequences. Children with a confirmed diagnosis of UTI are candidates for further imaging studies of the upper and lower urinary tract, including renal ultrasonography and voiding cystourethrography.

Recent research has demonstrated the significant health benefits of early identification and management of childhood urinary tract infections. Accurate and early diagnosis, combined with close medical supervision and improved health care, can minimize the long-term consequences of childhood UTI. Many effective and appropriate antimicrobial agents are available for treatment. Children with a history of UTI may require long-term,

low-dose antibiotic treatment until a full evaluation for anatomic abnormalities has been completed. If significant anatomic abnormalities are found, long-term, low-dose antibiotic therapy may be recommended for years.

Recurrent UTIs in children have been associated with scarring in the kidney, which may place children at greater risk of developing progressive kidney disease. Children with scarring in both kidneys have a more serious prognosis than those with scarring in one. Current investigations are exploring possible genetic predispositions for childhood UTI and scarred kidneys.

People with Urinary Catheters

Catheter-associated UTI is the most common institution-acquired infection, accounting for an estimated one million cases or more annually in U.S. hospitals and nursing homes. The medical and financial ramifications of this condition are significant: hospital-acquired UTI leads to one extra hospital day per patient, or nearly one million extra hospital days per year. Each episode of symptomatic UTI has been estimated to add $676 to the hospital bill, with catheter-related bacteremia, the presence of viable bacteria in the blood, estimated to cost nearly $2,900.

The duration of catheterization has been directly associated with the risk of UTI. Most catheterization is generally of short duration (less than 30 days) and is associated with hospitalizations for surgery or an acute illness. In contrast, long-term catheterization (more than 30 days) is often needed for persons who are in rehabilitation or long-term care facilities. Catheters enable small numbers of microorganisms that infect the urinary tract (uropathogens) to persist and multiply in the bladder in a short time period, resulting in an incidence of bacteriuria among people with catheters of 8 percent overall.

Virtually all people with long-term catheters experience bacteriuria, which is predominantly caused by as many as eight different species of microorganisms. Although *Escherischia coli* is still the predominant organism, these people are more commonly infected with uropathogens that are more likely to be resistant to common antimicrobials and more difficult to eradicate. These uropathogens include *Candida, Enterococcus, Pseudomonas aeruginosa, Klebsiella, Enterobacter,* and *Staphylococcus aureus. Proteus* spp. is associated with catheter obstruction in the bladder or kidney, renal stones, and chronic pyelonephritis.

Clinical ramifications of long-term catheterization include fevers, bacteremia, acute and chronic kidney infection, kidney stones, catheter obstruction, and death. Prevention of catheter-associated UTI depends on meticulous maintenance of the closed catheter system. Minimizing the duration of catheterization or using intermittent catheterization has been shown to significantly reduce the risk of institution-acquired infection.

People with Spinal Cord Injuries

UTIs are common among people with spinal cord injuries, most of whom are young men. UTIs in this population are often complicated and associated with significant morbidity and mortality. It has been estimated that nearly half of them will die of kidney-related problems.

People with spinal cord injuries have unique concerns that have an impact on the risk and management of UTI. Spinal cord injury can have anatomical and physiological consequences, including bladder over-distention, vesicoureteral reflux (reflux of urine from the bladder into the ureters during voiding), urinary stones, bacterial colonization of the perineum (the region between the anus and the vagina or scrotum), and high-pressure voiding.

> ### Spinal Cord Injury Risk Factors for UTI
>
> - *Reflux*
> - *Bladder over-distension*
> - *Urinary obstruction*
> - *Impaired voiding*
> - *Urinary stones*

The 1992 National Institute on Disability and Rehabilitation Research Consensus Conference examined the problems associated with UTI in persons with spinal cord injuries. The Consensus Conference report stated that indwelling catheters most likely lead to persistent bacteriuria, and, as a result, intermittent catheterization—although expensive and difficult to manage—is preferred. Intermittent catheterization has been shown to decrease lower urinary tract complications by reducing the incidence of stones, by maintaining low pressure within the bladder, and by eliminating the complications associated with an indwelling catheter.

> ### Pregnancy Risk Factors for UTI
>
> - *A history of UTIs*
> - *Lower socioeconomic status*
> - *Sickle-cell trait and anemia*
> - *Minimal medical care*
> - *Older age or increased number of births*

The UTI Consensus Conference determined that asymptomatic bacteriuria does not require treatment unless the upper urinary tract is at risk. Persons with spinal cord injuries who retain use of their hands, that is, people with lower level injuries or incomplete lesions, are more likely to be able to use intermittent catheterization, thereby reducing their risk of UTI.

At any time, approximately a third of people with spinal cord injuries have bacteriuria. *Escherichia coli* remains a common uropathogen, in addition to *Enterococcus, Pseudomonas,* and *Proteus mirabilis.* The presenting symptoms of UTI (particularly lower tract) in this population are atypical, and clinicians often find it difficult to determine when treatment is required. Clinicians with limited experience in managing persons with spinal cord injuries particularly tend to over-treat UTIs, thus increasing the risk of promoting multi-drug resistant bacteria.

Research is needed to provide further information about the transition from asymptomatic bacteriuria to symptomatic UTI and how to prevent this from occurring (i.e., method of catheterization, technique of catheter cleaning and changing, use of preventative medications, and bladder muscle pressure reduction). In addition, research should also explore why certain people are more susceptible to clinical UTI.

Pregnant Women

UTIs are the most common bacterial infections during pregnancy. From 4 percent to 10 percent of pregnant women will have bacteria present in the urine but will not have symptoms of infection (asymptomatic bacteriuria), and 1 percent to 4 percent will develop an acute UTI. Kidney infection or pyelonephritis develops in approximately one-third of pregnant women who have untreated bacteriuria, whereas bacteriuria rarely progresses to kidney infection in a woman who is not pregnant. Kidney infection is the most common, severe bacterial infection of pregnant women, and it frequently requires hospitalization.

Untreated, asymptomatic bacteriuria during pregnancy has significant consequences, including kidney infection, low-birth weight infants, anemia, and pregnancy-induced hypertension. Although some subsequent studies have disputed the earlier findings, untreated asymptomatic bacteriuria is clearly associated with acute kidney infection and low-birth weight infants. Research has highlighted the importance of screening for asymptomatic bacteriuria early in pregnancy. It has been recommended that pregnant women be screened during the first prenatal visit.

Elderly People

In the past decade, research has revealed important differences in UTIs between older and younger populations and within geriatric populations, depending on whether they live in the community or in institutions. A study of elderly people older than 65 years who were not institutionalized found genitourinary infections to be the second most common form of infection, accounting for nearly a quarter of all identified infections.

Symptomatic UTI is found among older men and older women and is generally considered to be complicated. Viable bacteria may be present in the blood (bacteremia), even without a demonstrable kidney infection. Functional and anatomic predispositions are common. Changes in the function of the prostate, for example, may predispose older men to UTI and obstructive disease. Neurologic and other diseases that cause incontinence and debility can increase the risk of UTI, and certain drugs such as antibiotics, anticholinergics (drugs antagonistic to parasympathetic nerve fibers), and psychotropics (drugs used to treat mental disorders) can have an impact on bladder function, creating conditions apparently favorable to UTI. Asymptomatic bacteriuria is a common and often benign disorder among elderly people, affecting approximately half of women and a third of men. Treatment of this condition appears to have minimal benefit in this population.

UTI symptoms are often atypical in older people and may mimic medical conditions such as pneumonia, heart attack, or dehydration. Older people are also infected with a broader spectrum of pathogenic organisms than younger people, and up to a third are infected with several organisms at a time. Antimicrobial resistance rates are greater among elderly people, particularly among those who reside in long-term care facilities. This has

Aging
Facts about UTI

- *As people age, symptomatic UTI becomes more common in men as well as in women*

- *Bacteria in the bladder can spread to the blood stream even before causing a kidney infection*

- *Symptoms of UTI are atypical; therefore, diagnosis is often made only after ruling out heart attack, pneumonia, or dehydration*

- *Resistance to antibiotics is increased*

been attributed to selection pressures in people who have been frequently treated with antibiotics or exposed to people who have been. Management approaches include longer courses of therapy (greater than seven days), preferably with fluoroquinolones or trimethoprim-sulfamethoxazole (TMP/SMX) when organisms responsive to treatment with TMP/SMX are isolated. In men, if the prostate is involved, longer courses of therapy may be indicated to reduce the risk of recurrence.

Estrogen deficiency in postmenopausal women has been associated with anatomic, mucosal, and smooth muscle changes, as well as with changes in vaginal flora. Older women may have anatomic changes that have resulted from childbearing or surgery of the reproductive organs. Topical estrogen has been shown to reduce the frequency of UTI by more than half. A recent randomized trial of women with heart disease showed no decrease in risk of UTI from one commonly used regimen of systemic estrogen. Because this trial was not population-based and other current regimens have not been tested, more data are needed before formulating recommendations for or against the use of systemic estrogens for prevention of UTI.

People with Diabetes

In general, people with diabetes appear to have up to four times the risk for bacteriuria than people who do not have diabetes. Bacteriuria and UTI are more common among women with diabetes than among men with the disease. In addition, persons with diabetes are more likely to develop UTI as a result of unusual pathogens that infect the urinary tract or to have severe complications such as emphysematous cystitis (an inflammation and infection of the bladder wall caused by gas-forming bacteria), and emphysematous pyelonephritis, which is the same type of infection but located within the kidney. Both diseases are diagnosed almost exclusively in people with diabetes.

The pathogenesis of UTI in persons with diabetes remains controversial. Underlying bladder dysfunction is a known risk factor for a subset of this population. Other risk factors include anatomical and functional abnormalities, poor blood sugar control, impaired leukocyte (white blood cell) function, vascular complications, and urinary tract problems caused by disorders of the nervous system. The microorganisms that cause UTI in people with diabetes are generally comparable to those that cause UTI in people without diabetes: *E. coli* appears to predominate, although research suggests an increasing role of *Klebsiella* and fungal pathogens in both hospital-acquired and community-acquired UTI.

People with diabetes, even though they may be ambulatory, are considered to have complicated infections; therefore, accurate diagnostic testing, including urine cultures before and after therapy, is important. People with diabetes are at risk for upper urinary tract involvement, obstruction, and severe or unusual complications, and they need to be carefully monitored. Imaging studies should be considered for those who require hospitalization.

Management of UTI in people with diabetes often requires a broad-spectrum agent and longer treatment durations (more than seven days for lower tract infection) because infections are more difficult to eradicate. Those who have kidney infections are often hospitalized.

> **Diabetes**
> **Facts about UTI**
>
> - *Diabetes significantly increases the risk for a UTI, and women are at even greater risk than men*
>
> - *Infections with unusual pathogens are more likely*
>
> - *Risk for severe and unusual complications of UTI, such as infection of the bladder and kidney by gas-forming bacteria, is increased*
>
> - *UTI is often the cause of hospitalizations*

People with Kidney Transplants

UTI is the most frequent infectious complication of a kidney transplant. UTI is also the most common cause of the spread of microorganisms and their toxins into the circulating blood (septicemia) after transplantation. Hospitalization is frequently required for kidney transplant recipients who contract septicemia because it is associated with substantially decreased survival. Factors that may put the kidney transplant recipient at increased risk for serious UTIs include bladder catheterization, immunosuppression, glucose intolerance, and short ureters.

Ethnic Populations

Few data exist on whether or not risks of UTI are higher in specific racial and ethnic minorities. Unpublished preliminary data suggest an increased risk of kidney infections in African American women.

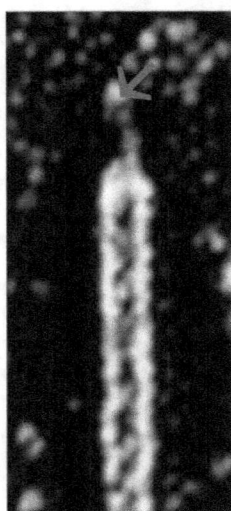

A high resolution micrograph of a type 1 *E. coli* pilus. The red arrow points to the FimH adhesin, which plays a role in the formation of biofilms. Biofilms cover bacterial populations, rendering them resistant to antimicrobials and antibiotics. *(Photo Credit: Matthew A. Mulvey, Joel D. Schilling, Juan J. Martinez, and Scott J. Hultgren. Proceedings of the National Academy of Sciences 97:16:8829-35. Copyright 2000, National Academy of Sciences, U.S.A.)*

Current Research

Recent research has made many gains in elucidating the mechanisms involved in the development of bacterial disease, the host response in inflammation and infection, and the innate response to infection.

Bacterial Pathogenesis

Attachment of bacteria to host tissues is a key aspect of the pathogenesis of UTIs. This attachment may be mediated by pili or fimbriae, by non-fimbrial virulence factors, and by other phenomena described below.

➡ **Pili (Fimbriae)**—Most pathogenic strains of the bacteria, *E. coli*, have filamentous projections on the surface called interchangeably "pili" or "fimbriae." The pili or fimbriae bind to specific receptors on epithelial cell membranes. As mediators of host-pathogen interactions, pili have long been regarded as important virulence factors in the pathogenesis of UTIs.

Type 1 pili and P fimbriae are most commonly associated with virulence in the urinary tract. Type 1 pili constitute a major virulence factor expressed by approximately 80 percent of common uropathogenic *E. coli* isolates. Type 1 pili bind to mannose groups on host cell glycoproteins. Although type 1-piliated uropathogenic *E. coli* bind to a variety of epithelial cells, including human vaginal cells, the specific receptors for type 1 pili on many tissues of the human urinary tract remain to be identified. In contrast to type 1 pili, P fimbriae bind to sequences in cell surface glycosphingolipids.

➡ **Non-pilus virulence determinants**—In addition to producing pili (fimbriae), uropathogenic *E. coli* produce virulence factors such as the secreted protein, hemolysin. This protein forms holes in cell membranes and induces changes in calcium levels within the host cells, possibly influencing cell signaling. Other examples of non-pilus virulence factors include cytotoxic necrotizing factor (CNF), which can alter cell shape, and Sat, a virulence factor associated with cytotoxic activity.

Often virulence determinants in bacteria are located on contiguous regions of DNA called "pathogenicity islands." Certain pathogenicity islands are correlated with virulence in the urinary tract. Since the pathogenicity islands are likely to encode other virulence factors, sequencing these pathogenicity islands, identifying novel virulence determinants, and understanding the functions of encoded proteins are key targets for future basic research on UTI. Subsequently, findings of basic studies may be translated into therapeutic advances.

→ **Internalization**—Laboratory studies have shown that epithelial cells in culture internalize isolates of uropathogenic *E. coli*. Studies in mice have identified a similar phenomenon in bladder tissue. These findings indicate that *E. coli* can establish a potential reservoir that permits intracellular proliferation of uropathogenic *E. coli* within bladder epithelial cells, and this may be the mechanism for recurrent UTIs. These observations generate many important questions, including,

- What is the nature of the intracellular compartment(s) or reservoirs exploited by uropathogenic *E. coli* in vivo (during infection in intact humans)?

- What are the mechanisms of establishment of these reservoirs?

- Are novel bacterial genes involved in intracellular proliferation?

- How do bacteria proliferate in such reservoirs?

- Are intracellular uropathogenic *E. coli* resistant to known anti-microbial therapies?

→ **Microbial dynamics**—Colonization of the vaginal mucosa by uropathogenic *E. coli* strains is a key event that precedes an ascending urinary tract infection. Yet in some women, the vaginal mucosa can become colonized without development of a urinary tract infection, or the UTI may develop weeks or months after colonization. The factors that promote the initiation of ascending infection from a colonization event are not yet clear, although bacterial responses to environmental conditions are likely mediators. For example, recent data indicate that a bacterial stress response pathway called Cpx regulates the expression of P fimbriae; therefore, virulence factor expression most likely can respond to cellular signals.

The expression of type 1 pili also is coordinately regulated by the expression of other virulence factors, and the adhesin of type 1 pili known as FimH plays a role in the formation of biofilms— collections of proteinaceous material (slime) that cover the bacterial populations and often render them resistant to sterilization and antimicrobial treatments. Thus, an important question is, how do uropathogenic *E. coli* modulate gene expression in the body during colonization and ascending infection? Quorum sensing is a mechanism by which many bacteria monitor their own population dynamics and modulate activity accordingly, and it is likely that uropathogenic *E. coli* employ a similar mechanism as well.

→ **Antimicrobial resistance**—One recent study showed that a significant percentage of microorganisms isolated in kidney infection were resistant to the drug, trimethoprim-sulfamethoxazole (TMP/SMX), resulting in a 50 percent failure rate for treatment of kidney infection caused by these resistant organisms. Similar, unpublished data from Israel on the treatment of uncomplicated UTI show equally high failure rates for treatment of TMP/SMX-resistant *E. coli*. These and other data demonstrate that resistance is a global trend. Thus, understanding the mechanisms of resistance will likely lead to the development of novel antimicrobial agents and extend the use of current therapies.

→ **Bacterial genomics**—Genomics is an increasingly important tool for the characterization of uropathogenic *E. coli* isolates. Related non-uropathogenic strains of *E. coli* have been sequenced in their entirety. A preliminary draft of the sequence for another strain is available.

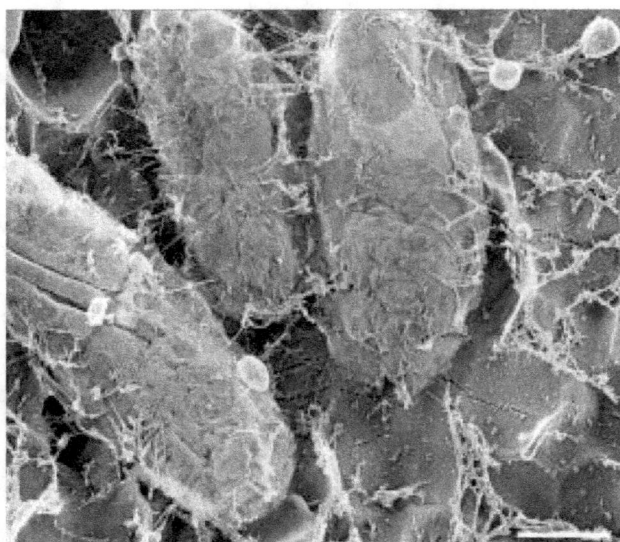

Type 1 piliated *Escherichia coli* attach to epithelial cells on the bladder wall. *(Photo Credit: Matthew A. Mulvey, Joel D. Schilling, Juan J. Martinez, and Scott J. Hultgren. Proceedings of the National Academy of Sciences. 2000; 97(16):8829-35. Copyright 2000, National Academy of Sciences, U.S.A.)*

Host Response: Inflammation and Inflammatory Response

The host immune response to infection involves discrimination between self and non-self, or between pathogen versus commensal organism, an organism that is harmless and actually benefits the species in which it lives. Immune responses are broadly classified as innate (natural) immunity or as adaptive (acquired) responses.

In innate immunity, host pattern recognition receptors recognize molecules expressed by the pathogen that are unique to it, highly conserved, and essential for its survival, such as lipopolysaccharide (LPS). In adaptive immune responses, lymphocytes recognize pathogens via specific antigen receptors, and memory for responses occurs. Innate responses are thus less specific, broader in spectrum, and present from birth without a known capacity for memory. Activation of the innate immune system may result in immediate killing of the pathogen and recruitment of adaptive responses, including elabo-

ration of cytokines, proteins that regulate the intensity and duration of the immune response, and other inflammatory mediators.

The connections between these two arms of the immune system are complex and the subject of intense research efforts. Although less research has been focused on the immune response as compared with other infection, some interesting recent discoveries have been made that suggest exciting avenues for further research. They are as follows:

➡ **Host response to type 1 pili**—The simple pilus-mediated interaction of uropathogenic *E. coli* with target epithelial cells can induce significant responses from the host. Type 1 pili induce rapid cell death (apoptotic response) that leads to the exfoliation (sloughing off) of superficial epithelial cells. This loss of superficial cells can be thought of as a host defense, since many of the invading uropathogenic *E. coli* are purged with the urine as the bladder lining is shed. However, the invading pathogens may also exploit the apoptotic (programmed cell death) response to establish reservoirs. Uropathogenic *E. coli* appear to actively enhance the programmed cell death response. Type 1 pili assist with the internalization of uropathogenic *E. coli* in a response that involves activation of signaling cascades and cytoskeletal rearrangements. How other virulence factors such as CNF1 interact with pilus-induced events is an important area of investigation.

➡ **Host response to P fimbriae**—P fimbriae also induce epithelial responses. In animal models and human studies, P fimbriae enhance urinary tract colonization, trigger the local host response, and lower the threshold for significant bacteriuria. P-fimbriated *E. coli* appear to activate the ceramide pathway via the release of ceramide from membrane receptor glycosphingolipids, rather than from sphingomyelin. Thus, while P fimbriae and type 1 pili share the ability to activate cellular response, they do so through different signaling pathways.

Cytokine production—Uropathogenic *E. coli* induce the release of cytokines from the urinary tract. Cytokines are hormone-like proteins that (1) regulate the intensity and duration of the immune response and (2) mediate cell-to-cell communication. Two cytokines, interleukin-6 and interleukin-8, are secreted into the urine at high concentrations. Epithelial cells locally secrete interleukin-8, a response that is important for the recruitment of neutrophils, a type of white blood cell, to the infection site. Uropathogenic *E. coli* elicit these cytokine responses when their surface molecules, such as lipopolysaccharides (LPS) and flagella, stimulate toll-like receptors on host epithelial cells. Interaction with toll-like receptors results in induction of transcription, which is mediated by NF kappa B, an activator of the interleukin-8 gene and a key regulator of inflammation. Uropathogenic *E. coli* can also suppress the activity of NF kappa B, thus potentially modifying host cytokine production. Other pathogenic bacteria alter the host immune response in this manner via specific virulence determinants. Investigating the means by which uropathogenic *E. coli* may suppress or augment host immune responses in this manner is an exciting new area of inquiry.

Innate immune response—The innate immune response to UTIs is thought to involve neutrophils and mast cells. Drawn to the infected bladder by the release of epithelial interleukin-8, neutrophils can act as phagocytes that ingest and digest uropathogenic *E. coli*. Mast cells, immune cells involved in allergic responses, are present in all layers of the bladder and are activated by interactions between type 1 pili and the CD48 glycolipid. This interaction results in both internalization of uropathogenic *E. coli* and activation of mast cells, which release histamine and other pro-inflammatory mediators. Although the potential role for mast cells in bacterial clearance from the bladder is not yet known, factors released by mast cell activation are consistent with the symptoms of bladder inflammation (cystitis), including pain.

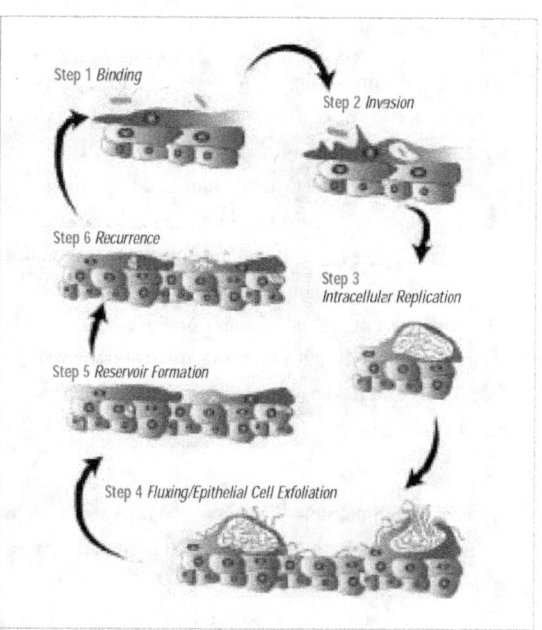

A six-step model of the pathogenic cascade of type 1-piliated uropathogenic *Escherichia coli*. **Step 1:** bacteria bind to superficial bladder epithelial cells through the use of the FimH adhesin on the tip of the pili. **Step 2:** bacteria invade the epithelium. **Step 3:** bacteria replicate within bladder epithelial cells. **Step 4:** bladder epithelial cells exfoliate and flux into urine. **Step 5:** bacteria form colonies and reservoirs in deeper layers of epithelium. **Step 6:** bacterial infection recurs. (*Photo Credit: Dr. Scott Hultgren, Department of Molecular Microbiology, Washington University in St. Louis, School of Medicine.*)

Research Opportunities

Opportunities for research into the cause, treatment, and prevention of urinary tract infection are numerous. Implementation of the latest tools offered by genomics and proteomics will likely contribute to major advances in our understanding of the pathogenesis of UTIs as well as identify novel therapeutic targets. Studies in molecular epidemiology, materials engineering (e.g., catheters), and vaccine development will help to identify susceptible people and prevent the occurrence of UTIs. Together, research into each of the areas described below will ultimately enhance our ability to prevent and treat UTIs and reduce this significant burden on our health care system.

Bacterial Attachment

Genomic techniques have begun to reveal intriguing, previously unknown, virulence determinants of E. coli. Emerging evidence shows that bacteria use multiple virulence factors to infect the bladder and that cross talk occurs between bacteria and host cells. In addition, bacterial resistance is rapidly emerging worldwide and has far greater clinical consequence in the urinary tract and beyond than previously understood. Key recent findings and intriguing leads in the areas of bacterial pathogenesis and host response to antimicrobials are summarized below.

➡ **Virulence determinants**—Bacterial attachment is thought to enhance virulence by promoting colonization of the urinary tract and by initiating effects upon the tissue, such as inducing the production of cytokines. Uropathogenic E. coli express several classes of adhesins that bind to specific receptors on epithelial cell membranes. The uropathogenic E. coli strain differs from most E. coli strains isolated from the feces of healthy people. Numerous epidemiologic studies have suggested that factors such as type 1 pili, afimbrial adhesins, hemolysin, aerobactin, capsule factor, and cytotoxic necrotizing factor (CNF) have a role in the pathogenesis of urinary tract infections. Many of these factors have not been proven to be involved in disease, but it is suspected that they contribute to the disease process. Furthermore, temporal control of type 1 pili expression may be required for successful colonization of the urinary tract.

Uropathogenic E. coli and other pathogenic E. coli harbor pathogenicity islands, large blocks of genes that do not appear in the E. coli normally found in feces. The pathogenicity islands possess genomes that are 20 percent larger than E. coli K-12 and other nonpathogenic fecal strains, suggesting the presence of many pathogenesis genes that have yet to be discovered. Genomic techniques are beginning to be used to discover genes present in a very potent uropathogenic E. coli strain but absent from an E. coli laboratory strain.

➡ **Type 1 pili**—Pili (fimbriae) present in most uropathogenic E. coli strains mediate the attachment of these microorganisms to bladder cells. Although type 1-piliated organisms induce the host to respond through programmed cell death (apoptosis) and the shedding of bladder epithelial cells, uropathogenic E. coli can resist the innate host inflammatory response by invading into deeper tissue.

The ability of type 1-piliated uropathogenic E. coli to invade the cells of the bladder epithelium and persist without being present in urine, may provide an explanation for some recurrent UTIs. One study showed that many recurrent UTIs are caused by the same bacterial strain isolated from the original infection. Research that proves uropathogenic E. coli is not strictly a pathogen that exists outside cells but one that could emerge from within a cell reservoir to cause recurrent UTIs would have a direct impact on the methods for detecting and treating UTIs. Studies that are currently underway to address these issues will eventually lead to new and better approaches for treating UTIs.

➡ **P fimbriae**—In animal models and human studies, P fimbriae (pili) enhance urinary tract colonization, trigger the local host response, and lower the threshold for significant bacteriuria. There is evidence for direct cell activation by specific P fimbrial binding glycosphingolipids (GSLs) and through disruption of GSL integrity and ceramide release. The exact mechanism of this process requires further study, but these data show that GSLs are important in cell-cell interactions and are involved in translating cell-activating signals. Additional studies show that P fimbriae recruit toll-like receptor 4 as a co-receptor in cell signaling, suggesting that the ceramide response is only one of several determinants of P fimbriae-mediated cell activation. Further elucidation of the effects of P fimbriae on cell signaling in the urinary tract will provide basic information about the function of this system, as well as a better understanding of a means of treating UTIs.

Host-Pathogen Interactions and Bacterial Pathogenesis

As compared with other pathogens such as *Salmonella* (typhoid-causing bacteria) and *Yersinia* (plague-causing bacteria), relatively little is known about how uropathogenic bacteria interact with urinary tract tissues to induce inflammation. New data suggest that uropathogenic *E. coli* cause changes in the bladder epithelial cells and cross talk occurs between them. Further investigations of these findings, as well as applying knowledge learned in other systems such as *Salmonella* and *Yersinia* pathogenesis, are among the key goals of future research investigations. These future investigations should

- Elucidate further the mechanisms of inducing inflammation and infection by known virulence determinants of uropathogenic *E. coli*, such as type 1 piliated and P fimbriated *E. coli*, hemolysin, cytotoxic necrotizing factor 1 (CNF-1), and others

- Coordinate regulation of virulence factor expression and pathogenic effects, including environmental sensing, host-pathogen cross-talk, and opportunities for non-antibiotic intervention

- Investigate pathogenicity islands and other undiscovered virulence-associated traits

- Conduct clinically based and animal model studies linked to basic science investigations in microbiology

- Identify other new pathogenic organisms of the urinary tract, possibly non-bacterial or fastidious

Genomics and Proteomics Technologies

To accelerate the discovery process in bladder infection and inflammation, infrastructures and initiatives in biotechnology supported by the National Institutes of Health (NIH) are essential to develop and employ state-of-the-art technologies, broadly including

- Microarray analysis for measuring gene activation

- Proteomics to determine levels of proteins

- Functional arrays to measure specific biochemical responses of epithelial cells and bacterial pathogens

Investigators would then exploit the high-throughput (the number of tests that can be performed in a given period of time) capabilities of these new technologies to rapidly analyze multitudes of clinical specimens as well as to completely characterize important experimental models of bladder diseases. These complimentary approaches would lead to an enhanced understanding of the pathogenesis of UTIs as well the identification of novel therapeutic targets for clinical intervention.

Molecular Epidemiology

New genetic fingerprinting techniques are under development and should be applied to expanded strain collections from populations of interest. Through the application of new and existing molecular epidemiology techniques, several key areas of research should be explored, including,

- Elucidation of the lineages of uropathogenic *E. coli* and other uropathogens

- Identification of the environmental reservoirs of these organisms (e.g., food, water, and animals) and the host

- Determine the means of acquisition and spread of uropathogens

- Characterize the development of mutations resulting in antimicrobial resistance

- Apply these findings to vulnerable groups, such as persons with spinal cord injuries

Knowledge derived from these studies can be correlated with findings from basic science and health outcomes studies. This will allow development of principles for controlling the spread of resistant and virulent organisms.

Host Susceptibility and Response

Research is needed on the following:

- Genetic predisposition and polymorphisms

- Existence of subtle defects and differences

- Innate and adaptive immunity in the urinary tract

- Chemokines, cytokines and their receptors, and antimicrobial peptides in the bladder and urogenital epithelium

- Individual variations in response

- Relationships of the host response with underlying diseases and comorbidities

- Response of the urinary epithelium to lipopolysaccharide (LPS) and other inflammatory mediators

Modeling

Small animal models have been useful in studies of knockout mice and specialized host response traits. Primate models might be more useful in studies of concepts that are specific to host and pathogen where primate host responses could be defined and compared with human host responses.

Vaccines for UTI

Two vaccines for urinary tract infections caused by *E. coli* are currently under development. The first vaccine targets the FimH adhesin molecule on type 1 pili of uropathogenic *E. coli*. FimH and type 1 pili are necessary for bladder colonization, and the vaccination that targets FimH on type 1 pili has produced protection against bacteriuria and cystitis in mice and monkeys. This vaccine also may protect against subsequent ascension of the bacterial infection to the kidney, since early studies have shown that the anti-FimH antibody prevents more than 90 percent of random *E. coli* UTI isolates from attaching to epithelial cells.

The second vaccine comprises multiple, heat-killed bacterial strains of *E. coli, Proteus, Klebsiella,* and *Enterococcus faecalis.* Currently undergoing Phase II investigations, this vaccine is administered as a vaginal suppository. Women initially receive one suppository per week for three weeks, followed by one suppository monthly. However, continuous boosters may be necessary, as UTI recurrences occur soon after treatment is stopped.

More research is needed to investigate

- Vaccines that protect against other organisms besides *E. coli*

- Vaccines that are not adhesin-based

Probiotics and Other Measures

Interest in alternative therapies has led to investigations of probiotics for the prevention of UTI. Probiotics are defined as living microorganisms that are administered to promote the health of the host by (1) treating or preventing infections caused by strains of pathogens or by (2) conferring upon the host other health benefits such as lowered cholesterol, reduced risk of cancer, and improved tolerance to lactose. Most probiotics are administered as food or dietary supplements, and benefits are assumed to be limited to the intestine.

Research has demonstrated that uropathogens replace the normal lactobacilli-dominant vaginal flora in healthy women who have UTI. In addition, a one-week course of the antibiotic, amoxicillin, was shown to disrupt the lactobacilli that normally inhabit the vagina. This disruption lasted up to six weeks. As a result, one proposed goal of therapeutic trials with probiotics has been to replenish the vaginal flora in people who have had UTIs and antibiotic therapy. This would be accomplished by the intravaginal application of exogenous lactobacilli. This avenue of prevention is currently under further investigation.

Another area of probiotics research is investigating the effectiveness of cranberry juice and other potential competitive inhibitors of adherence and colonization.

Future studies in this area will require the proper assessment of relevant outcomes, which are needed to better define the active ingredients in cranberry and other potentially inhibitory preparations.

Special Catheter Materials and Biofilms

Research should focus on developing special catheters resistant to biofilm formation that will reduce the incidence of infections in people who have indwelling catheters. Bioengineering collaborations to develop infection-resistant or antibiotic-impregnated catheters should be examined.

Health Surveillance and Outcomes

Current management of acute uncomplicated UTI is often empiric, without the use of a urine culture or of susceptibility testing to guide therapy. The rationale for this approach is based on the narrow and predictable spectrum of agents causing acute uncomplicated UTI and the susceptibility patterns of anticipated pathogens. However, as is true for other infections among people who are not in facilities such as hospitals or nursing homes, antimicrobial resistance among pathogens that cause community-acquired UTIs is increasing.

As the problem of antimicrobial resistance becomes more widespread, the use of narrow-spectrum, inexpensive antimicrobial agents becomes less feasible, affecting both the cost of, and the access to, health care. Preliminary data suggest that the increase in trimethoprim-sulfamethoxasole (TMP/SMX) resistance is associated with poorer bacteriologic and clinical outcomes when TMP/SMX is used for therapy.

Further research is needed to determine which factors best predict resistance and at what level resistance developed in the laboratory truly has clinical implications. In addition, surveillance data that combine susceptibility test results in the lab with epidemiologic and clinical patient characteristics are needed for a more accurate estimate of resistance rates among women with uncomplicated infection. Treatment of UTI may contribute to global development of antibiotic resistance.

Research Requirements

Workforce and Infrastructure

Multi centers and program research centers are needed. The National Institutes of Health (NIH) should also create new mechanisms and significantly modify ongoing programs in infection, inflammation, and interstitial cystitis to maximize recruitment, training, and career development of investigators in other disciplines. Possible mechanisms for achieving this include multidisciplinary training grants in inflammation, infection, and host-pathogen interactions and center grants or Centers of Excellence.

An NIH-Industry-Academia Task Force should also be established to foster interactive research with pharmaceutical and biotechnology companies in the investigation of UTI.

Tissue and Specimen Banks

The NIH should expand the support of programs that procure human tissues and bank them. In addition, bacterial and fungal isolates should be characterized so that they may serve cutting-edge research in infection, inflammation, and interstitial cystitis. The availability of a range of bacterial and fungal isolates and human tissues to establish DNA and RNA libraries should be ensured as well.

Advisory and Review Groups

The NIH should create ongoing review and advisory groups and public interest and educational efforts in collaboration with the National Bladder Foundation, the Bladder Health Council, and the American Foundation for Urologic Disease.

CHAPTER 10

UROLOGIC COMPLICATIONS OF DIABETES MELLITUS

Common Clinical Conditions

DID YOU KNOW?

→ Urinary tract infections are common in people who have diabetes.

→ Healthy post-menopausal women with type 2 diabetes have twice the risk of urinary tract infections than other women have.

→ Diabetes increases the severity of urinary tract infections and unusual consequences such as upper urinary tract diseases.

→ Peripheral neuropathy, a disorder of peripheral nerves and a complication of diabetes, can lead to increased amounts of urine left in the bladder after voiding—an environment that promotes bacterial growth.

Summary and Recommendations

Diabetes mellitus is a major health concern, and diseases of the lower urinary tract are common among men and women with both type 1 and type 2 diabetes. Because diabetes significantly alters the urinary tract, more than 25 percent of people who have this disease will develop costly and debilitating urologic complications. These complications include incontinence, infections, loss of sensation, and retention of urine. Unfortunately, the mechanisms involved are poorly understood. Moreover, little is known about the prevalence, natural history of progression, and risk factors of these complications. The paucity of knowledge has been a barrier to developing the best methods of prevention and treatment of urologic complications.

Clinical and basic science research projects on bladder and urethral dysfunction in persons with diabetes have received insufficient funding to make an impact on these problems. Only five basic projects and two clinical projects are currently funded at the National Institutes of Health (NIH). The National Institute of Diabetes and Digestive and Kidney Diseases (NIDDK) supports a number of ongoing clinical trials studying people with type 1 and type 2 diabetes and one population-based cohort study that includes adults with and without diabetes. These clinical trials analyze measures of lower urinary tract dysfunction, and they provide some beneficial information on urologic complications. However, ancillary studies such as these are often limited to self-reporting questionnaires, which provide information on the impact of disease on quality of life and activities of daily living; in-person interviews; and voiding diaries. These measures can only provide an initial broad view of urologic issues.

The Bladder Research Progress Review Group has concluded that new research initiatives are needed to improve knowledge of the basic disease mechanisms involved in urologic dysfunctions caused by diabetes. Research studies are needed to

⇨ **Improve methodologies for measuring bladder dysfunction.** Research must develop

- Urine, blood, or cell markers—characteristics or factors by which a cell or molecule can be recognized and identified—that are generic for early bladder dysfunction and useful in both clinical and animal settings

- Markers that are specific for diabetic bladder dysfunction and useful in both clinical and animal settings

- Neurophysiologic methods to assess diabetic sensory threshold and function

⇨ **Assess changes in the bladder and urethra that are secondary to diabetes.** To assess changes that occur in nerves, blood vessels, muscles, and epithelium, it will be necessary to

- Establish a formal link with Mouse Models of Diabetic Complications (MMDC) and other on-going studies to determine diabetic urologic pathology in mice, including urinary tract infection

- Study the effect of diabetes on female and male (i.e., prostate) urethral function

⇨ **Establish large multi-centered, randomized controlled trials of treatment outcomes in older persons with type 2 diabetes.** These trials will determine whether or not overactive bladder treatments, both behavioral and pharmacological, are efficacious in older men and women with type 2 diabetes. Clinical trials linked to other primary treatment studies should establish relationships between treatment and control of the primary diabetes signs and symptoms and incidence and progression of associated bladder and urethral changes.

Goals of Research

The BRPRG defined and described the following research goals:

⇨ **Clarify the basic disease mechanisms for bladder and urethral dysfunction in diabetes.** Conduct extensive further study of bladder and urethral dysfunction in diabetes to

- Identify and characterize the effects of diabetes mellitus on the nerves and muscles that contribute to urethral function, both during the filling and voiding phases of urination. Both *in vivo* and *in vitro* techniques should be considered to elucidate the mechanisms of action of diabetes on urethral function

- Perform biomechanical characterizations of both the normal and diabetic urethra

- Correlate changes in passive biomechanical properties and active urethral responses

- Evaluate the use of gene therapy to treat diabetes-induced urethral pathophysiology and, in so doing, develop new methods to treat diabetic urinary tract dysfunctions

⇨ **Identify the specific genetic determininants of diabetes and its complications.** Both type 1 and type 2 diabetes and their complications have strong genetic determinants. Defining the specific genes involved and characterizing the specific bladder and urethral manifestations of the genetic subtypes is essential to understanding the urologic complications of persons with diabetes. Examining these subtypes may allow preventive and management therapies to be tailored specifically to them.

Defining the genes for diabetes and its complications may isolate genetically determined environmental and pharmacologic response variations. Thus, a major goal for the coming decade must be to identify these predisposing genes. Collaboration with the National Consortium for the Study of the Genetics of Diabetes is necessary to create a strong, coordinated effort for analysis of the role of genetics in urologic complications of diabetes. Research should be enhanced in animal studies and clinical trials to discover the biochemical mechanisms by which diabetes genes function to create susceptibility to urologic complications

➡ Discover the disturbances in cell signaling and cell regulation that cause diabetes and its complications. Disturbances in cell signaling and cell regulation are central to disturbances in insulin secretion and action, which lead to diabetes and to complications in both small and large blood vessels. Basic research in this area is essential not only to understand diabetes, but also to understand many diabetes-related complications. Most importantly, this type of "discovery" research can identify important targets for new treatments. The NIH should

* Increase research in the fundamental science of cellular signaling as it relates to urologic complications in diabetes

* Expand support of interdisciplinary research to identify the mechanisms of these complications

➡ Develop a program to assess the effect of obesity on lower genitourinary tract function. Obesity is a major risk factor for the development of type 2 diabetes and insulin resistance, as well as a major cause of morbidity and mortality in the United States. Obesity disproportionately affects minorities. More than 60 percent of African American, Mexican American, and American Indian women meet the criteria of being overweight, and between 33 percent and 37 percent are obese. Moreover, obesity in children and adolescents is increasing at alarming rates, leading to the occurrence of type 2 diabetes in these groups. Obesity, including type 2 diabetes, has been causally related to certain urogenital diseases, including urinary incontinence and pelvic organ prolapse. Moreover, obesity and diabetes are described as factors that increase complications in those people

undergoing surgery. One mechanism to achieve this goal is to look at obesity as a concomitant but unrelated disease process in ongoing NIH-sponsored clinical trials such as those conducted by the Urinary Incontinence Treatment Network, Pelvic Floor Dysfunction Network, and Prostatitis and Interstitial Cystitis Treatment Network.

➡ Expand research into the complications of diabetes in small and large blood vessels. The different types of diabetes and the array of complications they present offer a wide range of specific research needs that are unique to each. The microvascular and macrovascular complications of diabetes are responsible for most of the morbidity and mortality in both type 1 and type 2 diabetes. Understanding and combating the complications of diabetes will require significantly expanded research on the mechanisms involved in the development of complications. Specifically, the NIH should

* Expand support of research to identify the mechanisms of the diabetes complications in small and large blood vessels that may relate to the lower urinary tract

* Recruit scientists from outside the field to enrich research on diabetic urologic complications

* Significantly increase the investment in fundamental research to determine the mechanisms of the nerve damage in diabetes, to expand research on nerve regeneration and rescue, and to evaluate methods to enhance peripheral and autonomic function

* Increase research to determine the mechanisms responsible for the loss of the vascular-protective effect in premenopausal diabetic women

➡ **Support research on the impact of diabetes in women, children, and the elderly.** Diabetes presents additional problems to women because of its impact on reproductive health and its causal relationship with vascular complications. Children and the elderly present special problems in the management of diabetes and may have additional physiological variables that must be addressed. To address these problems, the NIH should

- Increase basic and clinical research to identify the mechanisms by which the intrauterine environment, including the diabetic environment, affects both the immediate and long-term health outcomes for children and their risks of diabetes and obesity

- Support research to determine the impact of type 1 and type 2 diabetes on women, including the impact on their reproductive health

- Increase studies on age-related changes in the development of type 2 diabetes and its relationship to urologic diseases such as aging and pelvic organ prolapse

➡ **Increase research into the prevalence and impact of diabetes complications in minority populations.** Under-represented populations, including African Americans, Hispanics, American Indians, and Asians, have the highest incidence of diabetes and the highest rates of complications. These groups are rapidly growing segments of the population, and specific research must address the reasons for the disproportionate impact of diabetes that they bear. The NIH should

- Increase efforts in accurate identification of urologic complications of diabetes in minority populations

- Support research to identify risk factors, comorbidities, and primary and secondary prevention strategies for urologic complications of diabetes in minority populations

➡ **Explore the potential of genetic engineering for treating diabetes-related urologic dysfunction.** The ability to modify the function of cells through genetic engineering opens up tremendous opportunities for new therapeutic approaches to diabetes and its complications. The NIH should

- Increase research to explore the potential use of genetic engineering

- Bolster research to explore unique applications of gene therapy for tissue-specific approaches to urologic complications

➡ **Establish a comprehensive clinical research program.** This can be achieved through the following actions:

- Increase funding of meritorious clinical trials of emerging new therapies for urologic complications of diabetes

- Develop effective partnerships among the NIH, academia, and industry for collaboration and co-funding of clinical trials in diabetic urologic dysfunction

- Initiate clinical studies of promising new therapies for diabetic urologic diseases, such as gene therapy or tissue-specific approaches

- Initiate studies to determine the reasons that women and some minority populations with diabetes have higher risks for diabetic urologic complications

- Increase opportunities for, and support of, clinical research training

➡ **Create an infrastructure and develop resources that will enhance research into urologic dysfunctions related to diabetes.** An effective program of diabetes research can exist only if there is a supportive infrastructure. New and expanded initiatives are required to address issues such as human resources, clinical research, animal research, special needs, high-cost technology, and other components of infrastructure.

➡ **Establish mechanisms for the ongoing review, evaluation, and advice regarding implementation of the recommendations set forth by the Bladder Research Progress Review Group.** To accomplish this goal, the NIH should

- Create new mechanisms and significantly modify existing programs to maximize recruitment, research training, and research career development of diabetes investigators, including special initiatives to attract investigators from other disciplines

- Advocate and provide incentives for urologic input to the Comprehensive Diabetes Research Centers to provide enhanced infrastructure support and to enhance the effectiveness of existing Diabetes Centers

- Create a National Diabetes Technology Task Force with urologic representation

- Provide funding for assessing bladder and urethral function in collaboration with the Centers for Animal Models of Diabetes and Related Disorders

- Support mechanisms to develop and characterize larger animal models of type 1 and type 2 diabetes and their urologic complications

- Expand support of programs for procurement of human tissues and organs to serve cutting-edge diabetes research, to obtain appropriate tissues for the study of urologic complications of diabetes and genetic research, and to ensure the availability of a range of human tissues required to establish DNA and RNA libraries

- Establish an NIH-Industry-Academia Task Force, with urologic representation, to foster interactive research initiatives

- Establish a urologic advisory panel to review and make recommendations concerning intramural NIH diabetic urologic research efforts

- Advocate for urologic representation on Strategic Planning in Diabetes Research that would report biennially to Congress and to directors of the NIH and the NIDDK

Background

Although diabetes is known to significantly alter the urinary tract, the pathophysiologic mechanisms involved in this process are poorly understood. The best methods of prevention and treatment of these complications are also unknown.

Bladder and Urethral Dysfunction in Diabetes

Coordination of the smooth and striated urethral sphincteric mechanisms with bladder activity during urination is essential for efficient voiding. Diabetic bladder disease is well established, but little is known of the effects of diabetes mellitus on the urethra. Diabetes may interfere with both smooth and striated muscle relaxation at the level of the muscle layers themselves or at the level of the nerves controlling them. Indeed, diabetes has been reported to impair urethral relaxation in rabbits. This, together with anecdotal clinical evidence that men with both benign prostatic hyperplasia (BPH) and diabetes mellitus are especially at risk for urinary retention, suggests that diabetes may result in a disruption of vital bladder-urethral interaction leading to an increase in outlet resistance. The result is a worsening of the over-distension caused by the bladder muscle's weakened reflexes and its inability to contract sufficiently .

Sensory neuropathy is one of the most common complications of diabetes. The abnormal function of the bladder afferent nerve pathway (the pathway that sends nerve impulses to the central nervous system) is a key clinical manifestation in cellular disorders of the lower urinary tract that frequently occur in people who suffer from diabetes (diabetic cystopathy). Interestingly, recent research evidence has demonstrated that afferent pathways in the urethra normally play a role in the control of bladder function. This thereby leads to the possibility that positive feedback from the urethra's afferent nerves may also be compromised by diabetic neuropathy, the condition that results from the damaging effects of high blood sugar (hyperglycemia) on nerves. Such a situation would be expected to contribute to the weakened bladder reflexes associated with diabetes. Findings of urogenital afferent dysfunction in humans with diabetes support this hypothesis.

Epidemiology

More than 25 percent of people who have diabetes will develop urinary tract complications. Unfortunately, knowledge of the prevalence, natural history of progression, and risk factors of these urologic dysfunctions is inadequate. The annual costs of diabetes have been estimated at more than $98 billion. Approximately 16 million Americans, including more than 12 percent of adults older than age 40, have diabetes. In recent years, diabetes has become more prevalent in the U.S. population, and it is increasing as the population ages. According to National Diabetes Group Data 1995, type 2 diabetes accounts for approximately 90 percent of all cases of diabetes mellitus, and this subtype causes most complications.

As a result, in the next decade, a large percentage of the U.S. population will most likely have symptoms of lower urinary tract disorders. According to recent studies, diabetes appears to have the following effects on the bladder:

- Diminished sensibility

- Poor contractility

- Increased residual urine

Urologic dysfunctions such as urinary incontinence, urinary tract infections, lower urinary tract symptoms, sensory neuropathy, and urinary retention are common and costly complications of this disease. The epidemiology of urologic complications is not well known. In three large observational studies performed in 1990, 1995, and 1996, diabetes was reported to be associated with a 30 percent to 70 percent increased risk of urinary incontinence in women and men. Research on the type of incontinence associated with diabetes has been limited, but a study in 1997 suggests that the risk for urge incontinence increases about 50 percent, while risk for stress incontinence does not increase. Epidemiologic data are lacking on the prevalence of incontinence in men with diabetes and the relationship with prostatic hyperplasia.

Risk factors for urologic complications among adults with diabetes have not been well established. No clinical trials have been performed of interventions to reduce the risk of urologic diseases. And no prospective studies of early diabetic disease have included urologic diseases as an outcome.

Risk Factors for Urologic Diseases

Studies suggest that long duration, severe disease, poor glycemic control, and presence of peripheral neuropathy increase the risk of urologic diseases among adults with diabetes. One likely cause of urologic complications is microvascular disease (disease of small blood vessels), which causes damage to the small blood vessels and nerves of the urethral sphincter and bladder.

The metabolic consequence of intraneural hyperglycemia (high blood glucose within nerves) in people with poorly controlled or uncontrolled diabetes mellitus is glycosylation of nerve proteins, which leads to altered and impaired blood flow, oxidative stress, autoimmunity, and deprivation of nerve growth factors. Glycosylation may be involved in the pathogenesis of microvascular disease. Specifically, in diabetic rats, alteration in nerve regulation and dysfunction of the nerves of the autonomic nervous system result in bladder dysfunction.

The length of time a person has had diabetes, the baseline blood sugar (glucose) level, and the degree of control they have over blood glucose levels have an influence on new development and progression of other small blood vessel complications in persons with type 1 and type 2 diabetes. If microvascular complications also damage the blood vessels and nerves of the urethral sphincter and bladder, risk factors for microvascular disease may also be risk factors for urologic diseases among diabetics.

According to a 1998 study, certain racial and ethnic groups are at greater risk of developing diabetes than whites of a similar age; these groups include African Americans (1.6-fold), Mexican Americans (1.9-fold), other Hispanic/Latino Americans (2-fold), and American Indians and Alaskan Natives (2.8-fold). African American women, however, are at a three- to four-fold *decreased* risk of stress incontinence despite their having a higher risk of diabetes and obesity, which are risk factors for incontinence. No large studies have been conducted of prevalence for, or risk factors associated with, incontinence in different racial groups with diabetes.

Risk for Urinary Tract Infections

Although diabetes mellitus is commonly believed to confer an increased risk for many infections, especially urinary tract infections, data to support this are limited. However, in the past 30 years, several studies have reported that both bacteriuria (the presence of bacteria in the urine) and urinary tract infections (UTIs) are more common in persons with diabetes than in other people. Recently, healthy postmenopausal women with type 2 diabetes were found to have a nearly two-fold increased risk of UTIs. Most studies indicate that UTIs are more common among women who have diabetes than among men with the disease.

Studies have also shown that having diabetes increases the severity of UTIs and unusual manifestations such as upper urinary tract disease. Serious complications such as abscesses of the kidney or of the connective tissue and fat surrounding the kidney and decay of the kidney papillae are more frequently reported for persons with diabetes.

A number of factors have been postulated to increase the risk of UTIs in persons with diabetes. These factors include the possible effects of

- Glucose in the urine (glycosuria) and a high level of glucose in the circulating blood (hyperglycemia) on bacterial growth and immune function

- Peripheral neuropathy, a disorder of the nerves leading to the bladder that can cause an increase in residual urine volume, which can allow increased bacterial growth.

Few well-designed epidemiological studies correlating improved glycemic control with risk of UTIs and of upper tract disease have been reported.

Prevention and Treatment of Bladder Dysfunction

Control of blood glucose has been shown to reduce the risk of diabetic complications. Intensive glycemic control delays the onset and the progression of microvascular complications of diabetes, including non-inflammatory disease of the retina (retinopathy), kidney disease (nephropathy), and nervous system disorders (neuropathy) in both type 1 and type 2 diabetes. Reduced risk of large blood vessel complications such as atherosclerotic cardiovascular disease has not been clearly demonstrated. If small blood vessel complications are important in the etiology of urinary incontinence, intensive glycemic control may prevent or improve severity of urinary incontinence.

Weight reduction in women with impaired glucose tolerance decreases the risk of developing diabetes. Weight reduction in moderately obese women also significantly improves urinary incontinence. This improvement in incontinence in moderately obese women may motivate them to lose weight, which reduces the risk of developing diabetes, improves glycemic control, and reduces the incidence of small blood vessel complications. The long-term effects of weight loss on the incidence and severity of incontinence in women with diabetes has not been evaluated. Also, evidence regarding the effectiveness of weight loss to prevent or decrease diabetes or incontinence severity in different racial groups with diabetes is limited.

Direction of Epidemiological Research

Although urologic diseases are common health problems in men and women with diabetes, risk factors, patho-physiologic mechanisms, and possible interventions are not well understood. It is important to determine the following:

- Prevalence and incidence of urologic diseases for adults with type 1 and type 2 diabetes who live at home

- Risk factors associated with urologic diseases, especially aspects of diabetes severity (duration; treatment; glycemic control; and presence of microvascular complications, including retinopathy, nephropathy, and neuropathy) that are associated with greater risk or severity of urologic diseases

- Effectiveness of interventions, including glycemic control and weight reduction, in preventing or reducing severity of urologic diseases among adults with diabetes

Current Research

A review of the active research portfolio at the NIH has revealed that current research on urologic dysfunction caused by diabetes is limited. Although a few funded studies examine the mechanisms of bladder dysfunction in diabetes and the relationship to nitric oxide, insulin-like growth factors, and nerve growth factor, these mechanisms are not yet detailed. They have been conducted using diabetic rat models.

The NIDDK has a few prospective cohort studies among adults with impaired glucose tolerance, type 1 diabetes, and type 2 diabetes, and one population-based cohort study that includes adults with and without diabetes. Although analyzing measures of urologic dysfunction provides a highly efficient means of evaluating urinary incontinence prevalence, incidence, and risk factors among persons with diabetes, this area needs much more exploration.

The fields of urology and urogynecology have taken little notice of urologic dysfunctions in diabetes, and the work that has been done is mainly on clinical reports of urinary tract infections. More recently, there has been interest in erectile dysfunction in diabetes, with both clinical and basic animal model studies being performed. Reports are minimal on how diabetes affects urethral and prostate function.

Future Research

Objectives

The BRPRG recommends that scientific objectives of future research on the effects of diabetes on the lower urinary tract should be as follows:

- Identify and characterize the cellular and molecular changes that occur in diabetic lower urinary tract dysfunction and compare them with the normal bladder

- Develop short-term, clinical pilot studies to further characterize lower urinary tract dysfunction in persons with diabetes, and test novel treatment strategies

- Identify and characterize genetic markers that may predict early urinary tract involvement in diabetes

- Identify preventive strategies for diabetic complications in the lower urinary tract

- Determine the prevalence and natural history of urologic complications in longitudinal studies of men and women with diabetes

- Identify preventable or modifiable risk factors that will direct the design of trials to determine whether risk reduction results in lower incidence or severity of urinary incontinence, lower urinary tract symptoms, urinary tract infections, or diabetic bladder dysfunction

- Identify racial and ethnic differences in urologic complications

- Increase the diversity of scientific expertise applied to clinical and basic research studies of the urinary tract

- Integrate multidisciplinary groups of investigators to study urologic complications in diabetes

- Involve new investigators in research studies and training related to the urinary tract

Scope

The urinary bladder and urethra are complex organs with many interacting molecular, cellular, and tissue elements. The scope of the research strategy recommended in this paper is meant to encompass all the molecular and cellular components and interactions that occur both in the normal organ and tissue and in the diabetic tissue. Broad areas for investigation include, but are not limited to, the following:

- Pathogenic mechanisms

- Genetic mechanisms

- Therapeutic strategies

- Markers of early dysfunction

Stem Cells

Stem cells are multipotential progenitors capable of self-renewal and multi-lineage differentiation. They are, therefore, of great medical interest because of their potential therapeutic use for organ renewal and replacement. The BRPRG recommends that NIH launch a prospective study to identify and isolate multipotent stem cells or progenitor cells from the pancreas and to determine whether pancreatic stem cell therapy to cure diabetes can reverse the urologic complications of diabetes.

Research into urinary tract stem cell therapy should also be a priority because of potential implications for bladder renewal. Studies should be established to determine whether stem cell injection to the lower urinary tract can improve or reverse the complications of diabetes. Specific examples would be muscle-derived stem cells injected into the diabetic neuropathic bladder to improve contractility and stem-cell-aided *ex vivo* gene therapy to restore neurotrophic factors in diabetic neuropathy.

Research Requirements and Impediments

The BRPRG has defined needs in several areas that will be critical to advancing knowledge of urologic dysfunction in diabetes research initiatives. Manpower needs, infrastructure requirements, and the need for tissue and specimen banks must be addressed if this effort is to succeed.

Workforce

Only a few well-trained clinical researchers are investigating urologic dysfunctions in diabetes. A complete funding program is necessary to develop a cadre of well-trained clinical investigators and physician scientists. This program should include funding for fellows, young faculty, and mid-level faculty. At the young faculty level, funding for four to five years after fellowship (modeled after a K23 award) is necessary to allow for professional development. At the mid-career level, funding for four to five years (K24 funding) is needed for faculty to mentor fellows and young faculty. In addition, the program should give priority to the recruitment of quality scientists who have doctorates and expertise in diabetes and who would study the effects of diabetes on the lower urinary tract.

Infrastructure

Translation of basic research into human therapies depends on an active and vigorous clinical research program. However, several prevailing forces have significantly hampered clinical research and clinical trials in diabetes. Investigator-initiated clinical research is declining as a result of the

- Decreasing numbers of clinical investigators

- Limitations on funding of clinical research

- High cost of clinical research

- Complexity of clinical challenges

A major factor hampering clinical trials is the lack of infrastructure to organize and support them. A comprehensive program for tackling a significant public health problem such as diabetes requires a major investment of funds, not only in basic research, but also in clinical research and clinical trials. The latter are particularly needed to document the safety and efficacy of various therapeutic strategies and to generate the knowledge base for "evidence-based medicine" that will lead to better treatment of diseases. To achieve these goals, the NIH must

- Create an infrastructure to facilitate clinical trials—both to improve efficiency and to lower costs. This need is especially apparent in diabetes, where the path from clinical trials to "hard endpoints" may take many years and even decades.

- Commit to using clinical trials as a mechanism to develop the proper base of knowledge and to assure steady improvement in the care of people with diabetes.

- Establish collaborative research programs that would link bladder research with ongoing diabetes research programs.

Tissue and Specimen Banks

Tissue and specimen banking can serve the researcher by allowing single samples to be used in multiple projects and by allowing longitudinal collections with thorough source profiling. Tissue and specimen collections vary considerably from formal repositories to informal collections that reside in the laboratory freezers of individual researchers.

Urine and blood samples that may represent a reflection of bladder activity and offer potential for evaluation are part of a number of large, longitudinal studies. Of particular interest are studies that may allow the clinician to predict early diabetic urologic dysfunction. The following are either important longitudinal studies or NIDDK-sponsored studies with banks of tissues and specimens that relate to diabetes:

- Family Investigation of Nephropathy and Diabetes: serum, plasma, urine, DNA, and transformed cells

- Genome Scan for NIDDM Susceptibility Genes among Samoans: DNA

- Metabolic Epidemiology of Diabetes in Japanese Americans: white blood cells and DNA

- Diabetes and Cardiovascular Disease in Three Ethnic Groups: blood

- Epidemiology of Diabetes Interventions and Complications Study: blood, urine, serum, and DNA

- Cohort Registry of Type 1 Diabetes in Wisconsin: plasma

- Diabetes Prevention Program: serum and DNA

- Diabetes Prevention Trial for Type 1 Diabetes: serum, plasma, and DNA

Roger Parrish

Diabetic Bladder

Roger Parrish first learned that he had diabetes in 1994 when he was 55 years old. He was feeling extremely tired all the time and had developed bladder problems that caused urinary frequency and urgency. As Parrish tells it, "I was going to the bathroom to urinate about every half hour, even at night. I went that often whether I drank anything or not."

Parrish's physician gave him a complete physical and did a fasting blood sugar test—his blood glucose level was 720mg./dL, miles above the current threshold, 125 mg./dL, for identifying people with diabetes. With a diagnosis of type 2 diabetes, Parrish was placed on oral medications to lower his blood sugar and was given a diet to follow. After a few weeks on this regimen, he began to feel better, but the urinary frequency and urgency continued, although not as severe. He got up to void at least three to four times a night.

The elevated blood sugar in diabetes can cause autonomic diabetic neuropathy, a condition in which the autonomic nerves that help control the body's involuntary functions such as digestion and urination become damaged. Autonomic diabetic neuropathy (or cystopathy as it is called when it refers to the bladder alone) creates difficulty in knowing when the bladder is full, difficulty in emptying the bladder completely, and frequent bladder infections. In the latter, nerve damage prevents the bladder from emptying properly, and the urine that remains becomes a medium for bacterial growth.

Parrish's first urinary tract infection occurred not long after his diabetes was diagnosed, when he had a bout with gastroenteritis. "I felt like I was straining when I went to the bathroom," he says. "It was very painful." Urinary tract infections are rare in men but common in all persons with diabetes, as are other infections. "One of the biggest things that happen to you when you get diabetes is that you can suffer from more sickness,"

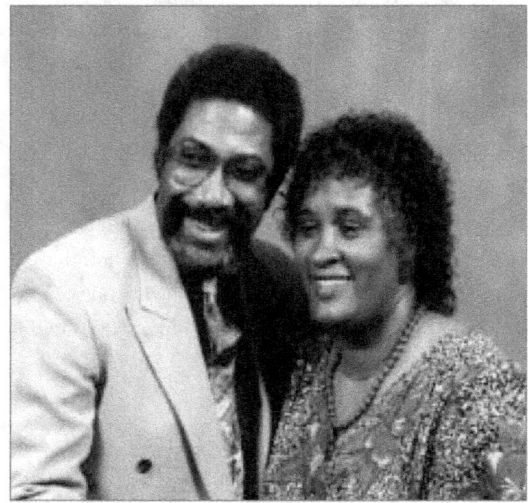

Roger and Frances Parrish

Parrish says. "Your system is more vulnerable and you get more bugs, more flu, more colds. I never had colds much before I got diabetes."

When blood glucose levels are maintained at a lower level, neuropathic symptoms lessen and may even prevent or delay the onset of other problems. Parrish maintained his glucose levels with diet and oral medications until this year when his blood sugar started to climb, and he developed other neuromuscular problems associated with diabetes.

In spring 2002, when he had surgery for a problem related to diabetes, Parrish developed a second urinary tract infection, which he says was precipitated by a drug reaction that occurred in hospital.

"It was very painful. I hurt more when I passed water than when I didn't, and it hurt worse at the end of passing water," he explains. "I thought back pain or a headache was pain but they didn't come close. It was terrible." Parrish says the infection had an effect on his blood sugar, which went up to 420 mg./dL. "I was lucky to have not suffered a stroke, which can happen when blood sugar is that high."

Parrish's urologist performed cystoscopic tests to determine the source of his bladder problems. A cystoscope allows the urologist to visualize the interior of the bladder and to perform tests that measure bladder capacity, elasticity, and contractility. "He filled up my bladder with a dye solution and it felt like I was going to explode," Parrish says. "It was very uncomfortable, but it was over quickly. I took pyridium [a medication that soothes the bladder lining] and antibiotics for months [for the bladder infection], and I've been feeling weak and drained. It drains you when you get an infection like that."

Parrish's physician recently placed him on insulin, and his blood glucose levels now range between 90 mg./dL and 146 mg./dL. The urinary frequency and urgency he had been experiencing have diminished considerably in the short time that he has been on insulin. He now goes to the bathroom every two hours and "once a night or sometimes twice." However, since the urgency diminished, he was able to hold his urine so well that he was putting off voiding when he was busy, something his physician discourages. "She told me that holding back too long could damage the bladder," he says. "It makes the bladder work harder and then it gets weaker."

Because of the severity of the urinary tract infection that occurred after surgery, Parrish has had to take extended sick leave from his job as supervisor of parking and transport at the University of Virginia where he handles special functions such as football games and conferences, and also from a part-time job as a certified nursing assistant at Martha Jefferson Home Health Care, where he specializes in the care of the elderly, a job that gives him great satisfaction. "I love being with older folks. There's a lot of wisdom and knowledge there," Parrish says.

Parrish might also be described as a person who possesses a great deal of wisdom and knowledge. Since developing diabetes, he has been particularly careful about his diet and lifestyle. Lifestyle factors such as smoking and alcohol can contribute to nerve damage in diabetics. A nonsmoker who also does not drink alcohol, Parrish believes this may have limited the severity of his problems. " My biggest problem had been eating and not getting enough rest. If I changed my diet 10 years before I was diagnosed with diabetes, I would have been better off," he says.

Knowing that diabetes was prevalent in his family might have helped as well. Although diabetes has affected almost every member of his father's family, Parrish never knew they had the disease until after he developed it himself. "Then everyone started talking about their problems, including bladder problems."

Parrish would like the medical community to see if there is a better way to educate people about the effects of diabetes and about how to prevent it. He also wonders whether research could develop a way to detect it earlier or prevent it and the neuropathy it causes. "Maybe some of the problems I had like the bladder infections could have been avoided," he says.

Parrish is trying to change the course of the disease in his own family by educating his children, ages 27 to 44, about diabetes and its consequences. Although he's had varying degrees of success with them, he says his wife has improved her diet considerably since his diabetes was diagnosed, and she stopped smoking a few years ago. The couple has enjoyed a long and happy marriage, during which they have taken memorable trips to various states and Canada and romantic interludes to the Caribbean Islands. They plan to stay healthy so that they can have more of the same, he says.

"I know I won't live forever, but I don't want to die for something I could have prevented," says Parrish, who measures his blood sugar three and sometimes four times a day, administers insulin accordingly, follows a prescribed diet, and sees his physician every three months.

CHAPTER 11

URINARY INCONTINENCE

Common Clinical Conditions

DID YOU KNOW?

→ Approximately 13 million Americans—many of them women—suffer from urinary incontinence, a condition that is not normal at any age.

→ Nearly half of those affected are too ashamed to discuss this problem—even with health care professionals.

→ As many as 30 percent of new mothers develop bladder control problems after giving birth.

→ An estimated 28 percent of adults over age 60 have some form of urinary incontinence.

Summary and Recommendations

For the 13 million people in the United States who live with urinary incontinence (UI), the condition is a daily embarrassment. Nearly half of these Americans are too ashamed to even discuss this problem with their health care professionals. Instead, they suffer silently, without help, becoming dependent on toilet paper, pads, or diapers. According to research studies, people who are incontinent seek help when their condition becomes severe, but many years of suffering have occurred before that time. Early treatment would be beneficial.

Most people afflicted with this condition are women. Despite the high prevalence and impact of UI, research has lagged significantly behind research into other conditions. In the current bladder research portfolio of the National Institutes of Health (NIH), UI research is under represented and under funded. It is a fertile area for development of high-yield research, with the likelihood of rapid translation to clinical care of millions of Americans.

New research initiatives must be launched to

- Improve understanding of the mechanisms of UI

- Develop more effective treatments

- Identify risk factors for incontinence and develop measures to eliminate or reduce them

- To achieve these goals, the Bladder Research Progress Review Group made the following recommendations:

⇨ Increase the size, scope, number, and funding for NIH-sponsored multidisciplinary urinary incontinence research centers

⇨ Encourage industry-NIH relationships in incontinence-related research

- Recruit established scientists from other relevant areas (e.g., cardiac or gastrointestinal physiology, cell signaling, biomechanical engineering, genomics, and proteomics) to apply their work to the urinary tract and incontinence by encouraging collaborative efforts between basic and clinical scientists

- Encourage special interest groups for conditions such as Parkinson's disease, multiple sclerosis, spinal cord injury, and diabetes to be advocates for urinary incontinence through better information for people with incontinence

- Increase research funding for studies that use cellular and molecular techniques to examine the basic mechanisms of bladder and urethral interactions that create urinary continence and incontinence

- Support research to develop appropriate animal models of urinary incontinence

- Develop novel techniques (both invasive and noninvasive) for measuring neural, muscular (striated and smooth), and vascular function relating to continence and incontinence

- Identify risk factors for urinary incontinence related to childbirth and aging so that prevention measures and improved disease-specific treatment can be developed

- Initiate research to develop preventive and therapeutic approaches to urinary incontinence that are sensitive to gender, race, and culture, and develop the means of measuring outcomes for treatments in these varied settings

- Develop a national data registry and tissue bank of people suffering from incontinence to meet the needs of researchers for well-characterized tissue samples

- Explore with the Centers for Disease Control and Prevention the possibility of establishing a national registry for surgical treatment of urinary incontinence, especially procedures using new technology

Background

Basic Mechanisms of Incontinence

The urinary bladder is a complex organ that is poorly understood at this time. It has a simple purpose—to hold and empty urine on demand. The bladder's function can be thought of as an equation of holding=emptying, with movement from holding to emptying routinely based on intentional neural and cerebral control. Incontinence therefore should be thought of as an imbalance—a tipping of the equation by one or more variables or by interaction of variables. There are many contributing components to each side of the equation—some more understood than others—but, undoubtedly, many variables are not appreciated at the present time.

HOLDING	EMPTYING
Bladder small muscle	Urethra small and striated muscle
Urethra small and striated muscle	Bladder small and striated muscle
Epithelium	Epithelium columnar and squamous
Hydrophobic interphase	
Nerves	Nerves
Neural transmitters	Neural transmitters
Growth factors	Growth factors
Collagen	Collagen
Vascularity	Vascularity
Hormones	Hormones
Pelvic attachments	

Some variables have functions on both sides of the equation. Historically, the most studied variable in UI—pelvic attachments—is a static one and pertains to stress incontinence, that is, hypermobility of the urethra. In fact, the most reproducibly successful solution for hypermobility is surgical reattachment. This success is predicated on an understanding of the underlying mechanism.

Our understanding of the basic mechanisms of incontinence needs to be expanded to include the complex biochemical and rapidly changing variables such as urothelial products—growth factors, collagen production, and angiogenesis, the development of new blood vessels, to name a few. Once this mechanism is understood, treatment development with translation to clinical care will follow.

Another example of a tip in the equation is the loss of estrogen in a postmenopausal woman. The bladder and the urethra are both affected by the estrogen deficiency, but the urethra's diminished vascularity and tone is more critical, resulting in incontinence and loss of control. Fortunately, once estrogen deficiency is diagnosed, treatment is inexpensive and effective.

The cause of a person's incontinence is often elusive. Currently, the medical community uses a small series of tests, including a physical exam, blood work, cystoscopy, urodynamics, and radiologic imaging, to evaluate a person who is incontinent. Each test gives reliable, meaningful, but limited, data. Estrogen deficiency will be determined by a combination of rather mild physical changes, nonspecific symptoms, and a blood test, which has only moderate sensitivity and specificity. More likely than not, a patient will receive an empiric trial. This is the state for many variables for the bladder equation detailed above. Many variables have no defined test with which to determine its level of effect on the bladder. Improved testing with yet-to-be-developed biomarker and imaging technologies is a major clinical need.

To successfully treat incontinence, the medical community needs to acquire a broad and in-depth understanding of the variables of the bladder equation along with their complex interactions. Studies of the mechanism of UI lay the groundwork for treatment development and rapid translation to the clinical care of millions of Americans.

Prevalence

Because it is a highly personal and often embarrassing issue, UI is far more prevalent than reported. According to some estimates, more than 13 million Americans suffer from UI, including 28 percent of adults above age 60 and 15 percent below. Every study that included both men and women in the study population has reported a higher prevalence of incontinence in women, with female to male ratios approximately 4:1 below age 60 and 2:1 for age 60 and above.

Established risk factors for both men and women include family history, impairment of mobility and cognition, lower urinary tract symptoms, and age. Some of the strongest epidemiologic risk factors in women include obesity, childbirth, and certain surgeries. In men, bladder outlet obstruction and prostate surgery are important risks factors. The frail elderly deserve special consideration because of the balance between co-existing conditions and bladder function.

Certain life events or health conditions increase the risk of UI. Urge incontinence is more common in women after they reach age 60, and stress incontinence more common in younger women. In women who have given birth vaginally, as many as 30 percent develop bladder control problems.

Some epidemiologic studies suggest that Caucasian women are more susceptible to UI than African American women (18 percent and 15 percent, respectively), and that Caucasian women have a higher prevalence of genuine stress incontinence compared with African American women.

Obesity is a significant independent risk factor for incontinence in older women. Some evidence suggests that obesity is an independent risk factor for certain sub-types of UI. Family history may play a role; first-degree relatives of elderly people with UI have been reported to have an increased prevalence of nocturnal enuresis. A similar familial predisposition has been reported for childhood enuresis.

In older Americans, UI has been associated with a 20 percent to 30 percent increased risk of falls and fractures and a three-fold increased risk of nursing home admissions. Although it does not necessarily lead to death, UI has a profound effect on the health, activities of daily living, and quality of life of older people.

Cost and Impact

The most recent estimate of the annual direct costs of UI in persons of all ages is $16 billion (1995 dollars). Of that amount, $11 billion were spent in the community and $5 billion in nursing homes. Previous estimates of UI costs were $6.6 billion (1984 dollars) and $10.3 billion (1987 dollars). This cost increase is greater than can be accounted for by medical inflation. Although costs of routine care, complications, diagnosis, and treatment are included, these comprehensive estimates most likely underestimate the societal cost of urinary incontinence because conservative assumptions about prevalence and cost were used.

The annual direct cost of incontinence is similar to the annual direct costs of other debilitating and some life-threatening diseases, including osteoporosis, Alzheimer's disease and other dementias, arthritis, and HIV/AIDS infections. While these illnesses vary in prevalence and in their effects on quality of life and daily functioning, this is a striking example of the large cost of illness of UI as compared with other common medical conditions.

More than 75 percent of UI costs are for the care of women. Costs for women over age 65 are almost two times the costs for women under age 65 (approximately $8 billion and $4 billion, respectively).

Risk Factors in Adult Women

Adult women bear a disproportionate burden of UI because UI occurs earlier in life and persists longer. Stress incontinence is the predominant type of UI in women younger than age 60; urge and mixed incontinence become more common after that age.

Childbirth is a known risk factor, and, according to most studies, the first birth appears to be associated with the greatest increase in risk. Vaginal delivery and hysterectomy are established risk factors for both transient postpartum UI and UI in later life. This association appears to be strongest for stress incontinence. According to some research studies, damage often occurs to nerves and muscles of the pelvic floor during these events.

Further studies are needed to identify modifiable risk factors of childbirth. Although risk of UI is not likely to have an impact on a woman's decision to bear children, and would not be considered an indication for a Caesarean section, specific events of childbirth need further investigation; these events include

- Use of forceps

- Type of anesthesia

- Administration of oxytocin (a hormone used to induce labor)

- Performance of elective episiotomy (surgical incision of the vulva to prevent laceration)

- Management of the second stage of childbirth

The complex interrelationship between events of childbirth, other reproductive factors, and the development of UI has been largely unexamined and is an important area for research. Gender-specific research is essential for advances in clinical care of persons with gender dimorphic conditions such as urinary incontinence.

In some studies, hysterectomy has been associated with increased risk of UI in women. Although the relationship may be seen because hysterectomy is a major life event for women, there is evidence that some subtle neurologic damage associated with hysterectomy may contribute to the development of UI. Continence surgery is not completely effective and researchers are diligently seeking better ways to select specific procedures for specific incontinent women.

Menopause traditionally has defined lower urinary tract changes caused by estrogen deficiency; however, data regarding the association between menopause and UI are conflicting. Several studies have even reported a higher prevalence of UI in older women taking hormone replacement therapy.

Obesity has been defined as an independent risk factor for UI in women according to one study. In theory, increased body weight increases abdominal pressure during exertion, thus increasing the amount of pressure on the bladder during such activities. It has been suggested that obesity is an independent risk factor for stress and mixed incontinence but not for urge incontinence. In one study, morbidly obese women who lost weight after barometric surgery improved their UI significantly. Research is needed to determine whether simple weight reduction in moderately obese women can achieve similar improvements in urinary incontinence.

According to some studies, family history of UI in a first-degree relative may increase the risk of UI three to six fold in women.

Risk Factors in Adult Men

Beginning in the sixth to seventh decades of life, the prevalence of urinary incontinence (UI) in men approaches that of women. Physiologic changes caused by increasing age (see Risk Factors with Advancing Age, below) contribute to this as does comorbid disease. Moreover, UI is the most devastating adverse outcome after treatment for both benign prostatic hypertrophy and prostate cancer. Both of these conditions are common diseases in this age group, with UI occurring in 1 percent to 5 percent depending on the type of operation. All types of prostatectomies ablate the proximal sphincter mechanism, which consists of the smooth muscle of the bladder neck and the proximal prostatic urethra, as well as the non-muscular elements of the walls of these structures. Although prostatectomy ideally leaves enough of the distal sphincteric mechanism intact to allow continence in the absence of bladder hyperactivity and sensory urgency, radical prostatectomy has great potential for significant distal sphincteric mechanism destruction. Transurethral prostatectomy is less likely to disturb this mechanism.

Overflow incontinence represents another form of bladder-related incontinence that seems to be more common in men than in women, although it occurs in both. Overflow incontinence results from obstruction of the bladder outlet or from inactivity of the detrusor muscle that is either neurologic or pharmacologic in origin. Overflow incontinence also results from inadvertent overdistention of the bladder. The primary pathophysiology of overflow incontinence is actually a failure of the bladder to empty. This leads to urinary retention with "overflow" incontinence caused by either continuous or episodic elevation of pressure within the bladder as opposed to the pressure in the urethra.

Risk Factors with Advancing Age

For a variety of reasons, UI becomes more prevalent with age. Even in the absence of disease, aging affects the lower urinary tract. People older than age 65 will suffer from UI—15 percent to 30 percent while living at home, 33 percent while living in an acute care setting, and 50 percent while living in a nursing home. Although providers and older people alike will dismiss UI as a normal part of aging, it is abnormal at any age.

Many physiologic changes occur to the bladder during aging, but these changes predispose people to UI—they do not cause it. These changes include a decline both in bladder contractility and in its capacity and ability to postpone voiding. In women, the urethral length and maximum urethral closing pressure also decline, while in men, the prostate enlarges causing obstruction. In addition, elderly people excrete most of their fluid intake at night; therefore, two trips to the bathroom at night are the norm. This predisposition and the increased likelihood that an older person will develop a comorbid disease (physiologic, pathologic, or pharmacologic) explain why elderly people are so likely to develop UI.

The role of impaired renal concentrating abilities, shifts in the pattern of fluid excretion to later in the day and night, slowed central nervous system processing and reaction time, and decreased vision and mobility and their interactions remain unclear. What is clear is that the complexity of urinary incontinence in elderly people warrants a unique approach as that which has been described in several medical journal review articles in recent years.

Unfortunately, even state-of-the-art approaches leave most older adults only partially treated. Moreover, criteria for the best use of diagnostic procedures in the elderly are lacking. Comparison of outcomes for different patient groups would be helpful, but outcome measures designed for younger people do not always weigh outcomes in a manner appropriate for elderly people. Further complicating the situation, older adults are more likely than younger adults to suffer adverse effects of both the UI and its treatment, and such effects often differ for younger patients (e.g., falling and fractures). All of these difficulties are magnified in the nearly two million Americans who are institutionalized, nearly two-thirds of whom are incontinent. Not surprisingly, the cost and burden of disease for elderly people living with UI are disproportionately high.

Risk Factors for Pediatric Incontinence

Although we are all born "incontinent," we readily learn to control when and where urine is passed during cultural "potty training." Some loss of urine control with urge is seen during bladder training, but enuresis or bedwetting is the main bladder control problem in children. Enuresis is prevalent in an estimated 15 percent to 20 percent of five-year-old children, and the spontaneous remission rate is approximately 15 percent annually between the ages of five and nineteen. The embarrassment and social stigma attached to enuresis is appreciable for these children.

Family history is an established risk factor. Other risk factors include behavioral disturbances, constipation, frequent nighttime voiding (nocturnal polyuria), depth of sleep, urinary tract infection, and spina bifida occulta and other neurologic conditions. The evaluation of enuresis distinguishes monosymptomatic nocturnal enuresis from enuresis associated with attention deficit disorder and hyperactivity disorder. Dysfunctional voiding and neuropathic bladder and sphincter dysfunction are the main indications for urodynamic studies. There

are urgent research priorities in the epidemiology of enureseis (properly classified), effectiveness of treatment modalities, and the prospective implications of childhood enuresis on adult UI.

Loss of urine in children other than enuresis should be termed urinary incontinence. However, less is known about the prevalence of this except in structural abnormalities such as epispadias and bladder exstrophy or neurologic conditions (e.g., myelomeningocele) that are associated with an open bladder neck. Many of these conditions are recognized and treated surgically. Otherwise, urge syndrome and urge incontinence in children may be treated with bladder retraining and biofeedback and the occasional use of medications.

Risk Factors for Neuropathic Incontinence

Because controlled bladder storage and emptying depend on an intact cerebospinal axis, nearly any neurologic injury or disease can lead to voiding dysfunction related to inadequate storage and uncoordinated emptying, and consequently to UI. Although normal bladder storage and emptying is based on low-pressure storage, neurologic damage may create high-pressure bladder storage, which may lead to subsequent damage to the upper urinary tract. Bladder and urethral dysfunction are commonly caused by stroke, Parkinson's disease, spinal cord injury, multiple sclerosis, diabetes, and disk disease.

➡ **Stroke.** Bladder symptoms are present during the acute phase in approximately 70 percent of stroke victims, and about one-third have persistent symptoms, usually bladder overactivity, urgency, and urge incontinence.

➡ **Parkinson's disease.** Voiding dysfunction is particularly troublesome in people who are afflicted with Parkinson's disease. Symptoms generally consist of urgency, frequency, nocturia, and urge incontinence. The most common urodynamic correlate is instability of the bladder muscle (detrusor hyperreflexia). Parkinson's disease complicates any consideration of treatment for prostatic enlargement, particularly whether prostatectomy will be beneficial or harmful. Men with Parkinson's disease and other degenerative disorders such as Shy-Drager syndrome often respond unpredictably to routine treatments.

→ **Spinal cord injury.** Controlled and coordinated bladder emptying depends on an intact neural axis. Loss of nerve input above the level of the sacrum (the level of the spinal cord responsible for control of the bladder) often results in lack of voluntary bladder storage and coordinated urethral relaxation and bladder emptying. This voiding dysfunction is often managed with intermittent urethral and bladder catheterization to empty the bladder, but loss of the low-pressure bladder storage capability between intermittent catheterizations often causes incontinence. Even with the best current management, which requires high maintenance and intense medical follow-up, people with spinal cord injuries are at risk for persistent incontinence and damage to their kidneys and bladder.

→ **Multiple sclerosis.** More than half of the people who have this disease complain of voiding symptoms at some time. In approximately 10 percent of people with MS, bladder involvement is part of the presenting symptom complex and constitutes the sole initial complaint, either in the form of acute urinary retention of an unknown cause or in the acute onset of involuntary bladder contractions with urgency and frequency. This instability of the bladder muscle that occurs with urge incontinence is the most commonly detected abnormality.

→ **Diabetes mellitus.** Peripheral and autonomic neuropathies are common in diabetes. Diabetic neuropathy has been attributed to loss of the myelin sheath that surrounds nerve fibers (segmental demyelinization) and impairment of nerve conduction. Middle-aged and elderly people with long-standing or poorly controlled diabetes tend to develop neuropathy, which affects the bladder as well as other parts of the body. An early manifestation of diabetic neuropathy may be instability of the bladder muscle. The insidious onset of impaired

bladder sensation can be the first manifestation of bladder muscle involvement. Surprisingly, few large, well-documented studies of voiding dysfunction in persons with diabetes have been published. The incidence of diabetic bladder involvement is uncertain, because people who are diabetic may not seek care for bladder symptoms. However, if specifically questioned by their clinicians, many report symptoms of voiding dysfunction.

→ **Disk disease.** Most disk protrusions compress the spinal roots in the disk interspaces of the lower lumbar and upper sacral areas of the vertebral column (i.e., L4 to L5 or L5 to S1). Voiding dysfunction caused by a prolapsed or herniated disk correlates with the usual clinical manifestations of low back pain radiating in a girdle-like fashion along the involved spinal root areas. The most consistent urodynamic finding is failure of the bladder muscle to have a reflex reaction even when full (detrusor areflexia) and retention. However, a herniated disk may initially irritate nerve roots and causes exaggerated reflexes (detrusor hyperreflexia) and urge incontinence. Surgical correction may not improve bladder function, and it may be difficult to separate changes in bladder function that are the result of the disk sequelae from changes that are secondary to the surgery. A prospective study assessing the bladder function of 20 elderly people after lumbar decompressive laminectomy for disk or spinal stenosis reported improved bladder function in 60 percent by one year.

Current Research

Research in UI is impeded by the lack of knowledge about the basic mechanisms of continence. Urinary incontinence is the least studied of all bladder conditions, and significant areas of study are absent or minimal in the current research portfolio at the. A review of the National Institutes of Health (NIH) portfolio found

- Little research on the urethra, even though experts have recommended that both the bladder and the urethra, which together form the lower urinary tract, be studied as a functional and anatomical unit

- Lack of age-, race-, and gender-specific urinary incontinence research. Anatomic, physiologic, and etiologic considerations clearly differ by age and sex

- UI research funding, moreover, fails to reflect the disproportionate majority of incontinence problems found in women and the need for preventing and managing these problems

Current epidemiologic research has focused on several life-events in women that appear to increase the risk for developing urinary incontinence. These unique life events include childbearing (especially vaginal delivery), hysterectomy, and menopause. New mothers who become incontinent are affected with urinary incontinence earlier in life and suffer longer. New mothers who have a single vaginal delivery have been estimated to have a two- to eleven-fold increase in the risk of urinary incontinence.

The NIH recently embarked on a major study that will investigate the nature of the disease mechanisms of UI. The Urinary Incontinence Treatment Network (UITN) comprises three clinical centers that will address a number of issues in the area of urinary incontinence, beginning with the effectiveness of current surgical therapies.

Research Opportunities

Scientific knowledge of the physiology of urinary incontinence (UI) lags far behind that of other conditions. Current understanding of UI may be compared to the state of knowledge about atherosclerotic heart disease in the 1950s. For progress to occur, future research must do the following:

- Clarify the mechanisms of incontinence so that better diagnostic tools can be made

- Identify risk factors that contribute to incontinence so that preventive measures and disease-specific treatments can be developed

- Define treatment outcomes

- Improve treatment

Basic Mechanisms of Incontinence

Research in UI has multiple potential pitfalls. Similar to cardiovascular health, a study of the system in its entirety (the lower urinary tract and its adjacent genital and intestinal systems) is essential for a sound scientific understanding of the development and decline in continence. The latter is currently dichotomized into bladder or urethral dysfunction, whereas most experts suspect that another mechanism might include neuromuscular dysfunction, anatomic displacement, or other defects.

Because our basic understanding of UI is inadequate, no good clinical tests exist to stratify and distinguish between types of UI. For example, one woman has urge incontinence because of a weak sphincter, another because of operant conditioning, another because of neurological damage, and yet another because of abnormal reflex activity or abnormal muscle reactivity. At this time, there are only a limited number of tests to distinguish between these types of UI.

Consequently, effective preventive strategies await a more adequate understanding of the causal factors. For example, the role of the maldevelopment of the urethra and pelvic floor, damage to the urethra and its nerve supply during vaginal delivery, and deterioration with age have not been studied. Studying the urethral sphincter, for example, in a woman who has stress incontinence because of the loss of urethral support reveals normal findings, while evaluating the urethral sphincter of a woman with normal support reveals important insights into the cause of the problem. Once this level of knowledge is reached, then studying the cellular mechanisms involved in sphincter dysfunction can proceed.

Risk Factors for Incontinence

We do not need additional prevalence studies. Current epidemiologic research has directed focus to several life events that appear to increase risk for development of UI. These unique life events are especially apparent in women. They include vaginal delivery, hysterectomy, and menopause. New mothers who become incontinent are affected with UI earlier in life and suffer for more years. Study of these vulnerable periods of life may improve understanding of these risk factors and potential interventions.

Prevention of UI and improved disease-specific treatment will depend on research that examines

- Development and maturation of bladder control in children and factors that alter this development

- Effect and impact of aging on the physiology of urinary continence and the interaction of age-related diseases, drug therapy, and lifestyle patterns such as habits

- Effect of risk factors such as vaginal delivery, occupational hazards (e.g., heavy lifting and restricted access to bathrooms), hysterectomy, menopause, obesity, race, prostatectomy, and benign prostatic hyperplasia

Clinical Assessment and Treatment

To improve clinical assessment and treatment of UI, research needs to

- Develop methodology to screen for UI in the primary care setting and quantify the severity of the problem

- Examine pelvic floor anatomy and physiology through advanced imaging techniques that will improve understanding and diagnosis of incontinence

- Devise testing that will differentiate between the different types of UI and improve or validate urodynamic testing

- Develop outcomes analysis to measure treatment efficacy related to continence, patient satisfaction, complications, and cost

- Develop and evaluate new surgical and pharmacologic treatments using these outcomes analyses

Research Requirements and Impediments

Requirements

The Bladder Research Progress Review Group has defined needs in several areas that will be critical to urinary incontinence research initiatives. Workforce needs, infrastructure requirements, implementation issues, and the need for other resources such as data analysis, tissue and specimen banks, and a system for reporting data must be addressed if this effort is to succeed.

➡ **Workforce.** The lack of clinical and basic science research in UI is a major concern. The state of knowledge for UI seriously lags behind the state of knowledge of other conditions. Yet such research has the potential to yield significant results, because so little is currently known. Poor funding, lack of scientific investigation, and stigma may have hindered the entry of researchers into this area in the past. Scientists with expertise in muscle physiology, smooth muscle pharmacology, anatomy, cell signaling, and neurophysiology are urgently needed to help elucidate the causes of UI. Attracting such scientists may require special funding initiatives in the basic science of this condition and education of investigators about the importance and prevalence of UI problems.

Workforce needs also exist in the clinical evaluation and treatment of UI. Primary care providers are the initial step in the evaluation and management of urinary incontinence in the community. Yet, many of these providers have had little or no training in UI, a barrier to effective treatment. Given the magnitude of the problem, emphasis should be placed on increasing UI education for medical students and primary care residents. Urologists and gynecologists are the clinicians principally involved in the specialized evaluation and management of UI, although some nurses, rehabilitation specialists, neurologists, geriatricians, family practitioners, and internists have a special emphasis and clinical interest in incontinence. A three-year joint fellowship in FlexiPlus Pelvic Muscle Rehabilitation System (FPMRS) is available to urologists and gynecologists through the joint efforts of the American Board of Obstetrics and Gynecology and the American Board of Urology.

➡️ **Infrastructure.** UI research may be especially appropriate for programs in multi-center networks and program research centers to conduct because UI is included in general pelvic floor disorders such as pelvic organ prolapse, fecal incontinence, and pelvic pain. The bladder cannot be considered an isolated organ in this system, and a multidisciplinary approach using urologists, gynecologists, coloproctologists, physical therapists, and pain specialists will best address these complex conditions. Program centers would be tremendously helpful in fostering such multidisciplinary interactions, especially centers with fellowship training. Multi-center approaches to research into the treatment of incontinence may solve some of the problems of research in this area. Multi-center networks in both non-surgical and surgical areas may overcome the problem of patient enrollment.

During the past few years, pharmaceutical and medical device companies have sponsored research in urinary incontinence because of the large populations affected by UI and the dirth of current treatment options. However, because outcomes analyses of UI are poorly developed, the measures of treatment efficacy related to continence, patient satisfaction, complications, and cost have often been incomplete. Through the development of better outcomes analyses and collaborative efforts, research of UI may be furthered more rapidly.

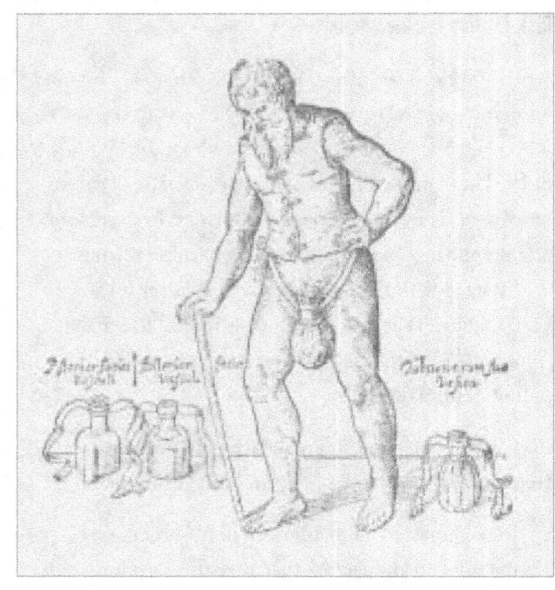

The enduring problem of incontinence. A 17th century drawing of a man with urinary incontinence. Around his waist is a belt with a bottle attached. In: Fabricius Hildamus G. Opera. Frankfurt: Dufour. 1682

➡️ **Implementation.** The NIH should provide strategically targeted requests for applications (RFAs) to initiate much-needed UI research that is consistent with the recommendations of the Bladder Research Progress Review Group. In addition, the NIH should investigate and facilitate study section infrastructure to facilitate proper grant review. Within the NIH, regular inter-institutional interaction and collaboration on UI research is also in order.

Furthermore, a program should be launched to educate legislators about the need for increased funding of UI research, which has been seriously under funded in the past. This discrepancy discriminates against new mothers, children (Chapter 5), and elderly citizens (Chapter 6) who disproportionately bear the burden of this condition.

➡ **Other resource needs.** Improving and expanding UI research will require the NIH to take the following measures:

- **Adopt the Consolidated Standards for Supporting Trials (CONSORT) system for comparing clinical trials**—The CONSORT system (http://www.consort-statement.org/) has facilitated the comparison between clinical trials in many areas and should be required in all NIH-sponsored clinical trials.

- **Establish tissue and specimen banks**—As in many areas of bladder research, there is a critical need for basic scientists to have adequate access to tissues and specimens for research. Genetic research can be advanced through the banking of blood specimens from well-characterized individuals in clinical trials. Once genetic determinants of UI are identified, these specimens can be used to amplify the knowledge obtained in small genetic studies.

- **Analyze cost, outcomes, and preference data**—Cost-effectiveness analyses incorporate data on both health care outcomes and costs. These analyses comprehensively describe the relative value of alternative interventions for a specific medical condition. For UI, cost-effectiveness analyses have focused on strategies for nursing home management and on comparison of surgical techniques for stress incontinence. Few data are available on the costs or cost-effectiveness of behavioral or surgical treatments. No data are available on patient preference (utility) for treatment and health outcomes in UI.

Impediments

Several impediments to research exist as well, which must be corrected if research outcomes are to be favorable. Those impediments include limited UI experience in review groups, the presence of concomitant but unrelated disease processes (comorbidities), and a social stigma that precludes the formation of an effective lobbying group for people who suffer from UI.

➡ **Limited UI expertise in grant review groups.** As the NIH is currently structured, multiple study sections review requests for funding of UI research; expertise in UI is not required for membership in these study sections. There is a need for inter-institution NIH synergies and for RFAs in UI to be reviewed by *ad hoc* study sections with experts in urinary incontinence.

➡ **Comorbidities.** Concomitant but unrelated pathologic or disease processes (comorbidities) complicate UI research. Comorbidities in the pelvis that need to be considered include disease of the prostate, aging, pelvic organ prolapse, pelvic pain, fecal incontinence, and rectal prolapse. Comorbidities outside the urinary tract must be considered as well; they include systemic disease, diabetes, and neurologic disorders.

➡ **Social stigma and lack of an active lobbying group.** Another important impediment to UI research is the stigma attached to the condition. Although millions of Americans suffer from UI, they are too embarrassed to come forward to publicly discuss their problem. This stigma has been a significant barrier to research funding and participation in clinical trials because people with UI have not formed active lobbying or advocacy groups. As a result, even experienced legislators are not aware of the scope of UI and the suffering it causes. Research funding is also often enhanced when a public figure discusses the personal effects of a condition. To date, no public figure has been willing to discuss his or her personal struggles with UI.

Melissa Lavender

Pelvic Floor Trauma, Incontinence

Melissa Lavender got out of bed the morning after her first child was born and realized that she had "no bladder control at all." Until then, she had led an active life with no medical problems to speak of. She watched her diet. She jogged 12 miles a week. She exercised to keep her muscles toned.

Lavender who was 40 when her son was born had had the choice during labor of having a Cesarean section or a vaginal delivery with the assistance of forceps. She chose the latter, but now believes that her bladder problems were the result of that choice. In fact, childbirth in any form is a known risk factor, and, according to most studies, the first birth appears to be associated with the greatest increase in risk. Trauma to the muscles and nerves of the pelvic floor during childbirth—such as that which can occur during prolonged pushing—can result in incontinence during the postpartum period, and it places a woman at a greater risk for incontinence later in life.

During the weeks that followed childbirth, Lavender struggled to balance her new role as a mother with the challenges presented by her physical condition. She felt that in time, the incontinence would improve, but it continued to be severe. At her six-week exam, Lavender sought the advice of her obstetrician/gynecologist, who told her to wait six months because research studies indicate that if the problem is minor, it goes away in that time. The physician also prescribed Kegel exercises to strengthen the pelvic floor muscles. Lavender performed them regularly, but at the end of three months, her condition had not improved.

Lavender then decided to consult a physician who specializes in the urologic as well as the gynecologic problems of women. "She was very empathic," Lavender says. "She told me that my pelvic floor muscles were, in effect, in shock and not functioning properly due to the traumatic procedure."

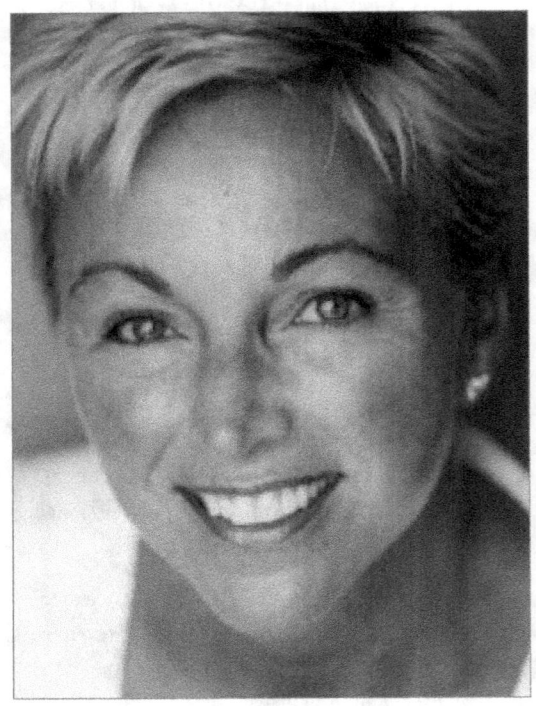

The physician gave her a pessary, an appliance that supports the uterus and corrects displacement, and an electronic device that stimulates muscles to improve tone. Lavender used both, and the stimulator did improve muscle tone in the pelvic floor, but the improvement lasted only as long as she used the device. Lavender longed to return to her normal life. She wanted to run again, she wanted to return to the satisfying sexual relationship she had had with her husband, and she wanted another child.

"Incontinence wreaks havoc on your life," she says. "I felt unattractive and unappealing. It stressed my sexual relationship with my husband even though he reassured me that everything was fine. I was depressed and always felt that I could smell urine. I wore pads all the time, and they got thicker. Any bearing down motion like bending over to pick something up from the floor caused leakage. Eventually, I got good enough so I could manage a run, but I had to plan it so that there was a bathroom midway. Women who suffer incontinence are always aware of where the bathroom is."

Lavender decided to consult a physical therapist specializing in pelvic floor dysfunction. She learned to plan her trips to the bathroom rather than urinating on demand; she learned the proper way to perform Kegel exercises and was given an exercise program. "Proper pelvic floor exercises and bladder training are very hard to do," Lavender says. "But I got to the point of dealing with the incontinence as many people do."

The incontinence eventually improved, but when Lavender became pregnant again, her bladder problems returned, and they were worse. In April 2001, she gave birth to her second child, a daughter, and the delivery went well, but she continued to be incontinent. She used more absorbent pads and did bladder training again, but did not sufficiently improve.

Eight months later, Lavender had a hysterectomy, surgical reconstruction of the vagina, and a procedure to "tack up" the urethra and bladder. After surgery, she followed a 12-week protocol—no lifting (not even the baby)—which necessitated household help 24 hours a day, seven days a week—and no sexual relations. Nine weeks later, she says she was 75 percent better.

"I've come to realize that there is no happy pill. If this is as good as it gets, at least I'm better," Lavender says. "I'm trying to go to the bathroom every one and a half hours. It's still challenging to make it to the toilet when I have to go. I'm also doing a structured set of Kegel exercises, and probably eventually will use a muscle stimulator again. I watch my diet, and constipation is forbidden…. I'm aware of my condition all the time."

Lavender has become an advocate for women's health, particularly for women who suffer from urinary incontinence. She is especially concerned about the stigma attached to incontinence. "Thirteen to twenty million women are incontinent, but no one talks about it," she says. "People talk about sex all the time on television, but incontinence—no one goes there. No one wants to wear a little yellow ribbon. This isn't something we should carry about in our own little world."

For the time being, she has confined her initiatives to the Chicago area. She is starting support groups for women with incontinence who are postpartum, menopausal, and elderly and is working on monthly education forums at local hospitals. She has also launched a publicity campaign to encourage people who have incontinence to talk about how it has affected the quality of their lives.

"It's tragic that we don't even know how many people have this problem because people aren't talking about it," she says. "If we don't talk about it, nothing will be done."

CHAPTER 12

URETHELIAL CANCER (BLADDER CANCER)

Common Clinical Conditions

DID YOU KNOW?

→ Bladder cancer is the fifth most commonly diagnosed, non-skin malignancy in Americans.

→ Bladder cancer is closely associated with environmental toxins.

→ Approximately 400,000 people had bladder cancer in 1999.

→ Men have four times the rate of bladder cancer of women.

→ Women and African Americans of both genders have a 35 percent to 100 percent greater likelihood of dying from bladder cancer if they develop it than Caucasian men do.

Summary and Recommendations

As people age, incidence and mortality from bladder cancer increase. Both incidence and disease-specific mortality are roughly twice as great for men and women after age 80 than they are for men and women ages 65 to 69. People with bladder cancer require numerous treatments that are highly morbid, expensive, and time-intensive (even for monitoring indolent disease), and family members or society must often assume these expenses, particularly for home care and transportation.

The impact of bladder cancer is greatest in middle-aged and elderly Caucasian men. It is the seventh leading cause of cancer death in men and the fifth most commonly diagnosed, non-cutaneous malignancy in the United States. Approximately 12,000 Americans die each year from bladder cancer according to the National Cancer Institute. Based strictly on these factors alone, both the financial and societal costs of bladder cancer are considerable.

The Bladder Research Progress Review Group divided research priorities for urothelial cancer into two levels.

Level I Priorities

→ Develop early detection, prevention, and chemoprevention techniques

→ Develop models (including animal models) of prevention, abnormal growth regulation, differentiation, and control to assess field effect versus clonality and to define urothelial alterations that are associated with age and gender

→ Investigate the basic biology of urothelial cancer, including growth factors, cell signaling, development of new blood vessels (angiogenesis), wound healing, programmed cell death (apoptosis), and cell-cell interactions

→ Study and implement strategies to reverse the dramatic gender, race, and age disparities that currently exist

Create a research infrastructure by establishing

- Tissue banks

- Specimen arrays

- cDNA microarrays

- Proteomics with demographic, clinical, and outcome correlation

- Matched and unmatched normal specimens

- Informatics and mathematical systems to analyze data, model applications, and future studies

Create a research infrastructure by instituting multidisciplinary collaborative grants and training opportunities to enhance team building and attract new investigators to the field

Level II Priorities

Improve and develop imaging techniques such as

- Virtual endoscopy

- Contact microscopy

- Fluorescent cystoscopy

- Novel ultrasound examinations

- Magnetic resonance imaging (MRI)

- Positron emissions tomography (PET)

Develop and improve gene delivery to the urothelium

Background

About 400,000 Americans have been estimated to have epithelial cancer of the bladder (urothelial cancer). Because urothelial cancer is almost never found incidentally at autopsy, and because the means of diagnosis—endoscopic inspection and biopsy—have not changed for many decades, this increased incidence cannot be attributed to improvements in diagnostic methods such as technological innovations or changes in health practice (e.g., organized or *ad lib* screening).

Epidemiology

Several characteristics of urothelial cancer make it particularly suitable for epidemiological investigations. Of all the urologic malignancies, urothelial cancer is most closely associated with environmental carcinogens. Several putative carcinogenic exposures have been identified in humans, including

- Cigarette smoke

- A variety of industrial and workplace exposures

- Arsenic and other chemicals in artesian well water in endemic regions of blackfoot disease in Taiwan, Chile, and Argentina

- Chinese weight reduction herbs contaminated by *A. franghi*

- Acetaminophen and other analgesics

- Chronic, continual urinary tract infections—particularly infections of *S. hematobium* or infections occurring in patients with bladders that have been damaged because of events originating in the nervous system (neurogenic bladders) and indwelling catheters

The demographic profile of urothelial cancer is well characterized, being most common in middle-aged and elderly Caucasian men in the United States. Men have four times the rate of women. Women and African Americans of both genders have roughly one-third to one-half the incidence of this cancer than Caucasian men, but these two groups have a 35 percent to 100 percent greater likelihood of dying from bladder cancer than white men do if they develop it. Understanding these differences quite likely will at least "level the playing field" by normalizing mortality rates to those of middle-aged Caucasian men.

As people age, incidence of and mortality from bladder cancer increase. Incidence for both men and women roughly doubles between ages 65 and 69 and after age 80. Moreover, if bladder cancer develops after age 80, the chance of dying from it also doubles. These differences are unquestionably caused by many factors, which include

- Specific characteristics of tumor biology and host defenses

- Personal, societal, and group values that influence habits, lifestyles, and patterns of behavior

- Availability of health care

- Concomitant but unrelated disease processes (comorbidities) that influence diagnostic evaluations, management recommendations, and treatments selected, as well as other factors

A comprehensive investigation of these issues has not been carried out.

According to biological and clinical trial evidence, early detection may be beneficial in reducing mortality and morbidity from this disease, although a prospective randomized screening study with unscreened controls has never been carried out. Of great relevance to the screening issue is that urothelial cancer is almost never found incidentally at autopsy, implying that early detection in asymptomatic people is not likely to be harmful. Additionally, this means that the repetitions of testing must be relatively frequent because the pre-clinical prevalence of bladder cancer is quite brief.

Finally, although the methods of genetic fingerprinting are improving and more information is being obtained about genetic influences that control inactivation and activation of several putative carcinogenic agents in the environment, compelling data to demonstrate the existence of a major inherited susceptibility for this disease are lacking. Indeed, the little data that do exist indicate that, except for extremely rare cases associated with an obvious familial predisposition, strong inherited tendencies are not seen. These data highlight the need for further understanding of the multitudinous events taking part in the development of bladder cancer.

Cost of Bladder Cancer

The therapies used to treat aggressive, localized, and metastatic disease include surgical removal of the bladder and urinary diversion, high-dose pelvic radiotherapy, and multi-drug chemotherapy. These therapies are highly morbid and expensive. Urothelial cancer is the second most prevalent malignancy in middle-aged and elderly men, who must undergo continued surveillance examinations that are costly and somewhat morbid. Precise economic assessments of these exams are needed.

Based on at least preliminary analyses, screening for bladder cancer would be cost-effective when compared with other diseases where early detection has been recognized as beneficial (e.g., mammography for breast cancer and blood pressure checks for hypertension). Because our understanding of bladder cancer biology is limited and the treatments for aggressive local, regional, and metastatic disease are still not very effective and are associated with significant morbidities, the potentially positive impact of early intervention on reducing mortality at a seemingly acceptable economic cost would be important to investigate.

Because bladder cancer is primarily a disease of the elderly, with the median age at diagnosis for both men and women being well beyond the usual age of retirement, cancer of the bladder and its treatment may at first seem to have relatively little impact on economic productivity. However, people with this disease require numerous treatments that are time-intensive (even for monitoring indolent disease), and family members or society must often assume these expenses, particularly for home care and transportation. Thus, sophisticated economic analyses are needed to remotely understand not only the direct health care costs of this disease, but also the societal costs.

Impact of Bladder Cancer

When urothelial cancer invades bladder muscle, the standard treatment for locally invasive cancer remains surgical removal of the bladder (cystectomy) and some form of urinary diversion. Although in healthy people, a high proportion of men and a significant proportion of women can undergo orthotopic bladder substitution (substitution in the normal position of the bladder), this situation is not the same as having one's own bladder. Under the best of circumstances, urinations are not normal; roughly 80 percent of those who have had substitution wake up at night to urinate (nocturia) or experience nocturnal incontinence, 5 percent or more experience daytime stress incontinence, and 20 percent to 30 percent of women have urinary retention that requires intermittent self-catheterization.

Additionally, the instances of urinary tract infections and upper urinary tract compromise are certainly greater than when a normal bladder is in place. Depending on the patient's desires, the comorbidities involved, the extent of the tumor, and the technical considerations, approximately 25 percent to 50 percent of men and 50 percent to 75 percent of women who undergo cystectomy cannot undergo bladder substitution. Although both continent, catheterizable reservoirs and conduit systems to handle diverted urine are technically quite successful, their psychological and physical impact may be negative because a small abdominal opening called a stoma is necessary. Abdominal stomas are also associated with a high incidence of urinary tract infections and upper urinary tract deterioration.

Short-term voiding function complications caused by pelvic radiotherapy tend to be less than those caused by a cystectomy. However, at least 5 percent to 10 percent of patients experience significant long-term bladder or rectal toxicities, which can range from being manageable

annoyances to life-threatening matters. Surgical treatments for the latter often have extremely serious consequences. Thus, a comprehensive assessment is needed of the consequences of urothelial cancer treatment, particularly its effects on the bladder's function(s) over time.

> ### Orthotopic Bladder Substitution: Complications
>
> * *Bedwetting*
> * *Night-time voiding*
> * *Stress incontinence*
> * *Urinary retention*
> * *Urinary tract infection*

Significant sexual problems also result from bladder cancer therapies. The vagina of women treated by either cystectomy or radiation therapy often becomes nearly functionless because its size is compromised, lubrication is inadequate, and the formation of fibrous tissue (fibrosis) has occurred (particularly after radiation), making it inelastic. In certain women, this is a major issue. Men, despite the employment of nerve-sparing surgical techniques, experience at least a 30 percent to 40 percent chance of serious erectile dysfunction, depending on their age, comorbidities, and smoking exposure. If anything but a thorough attempt is made to spare nerves controlling erections or if a total removal of the urethra (urethrectomy) is needed, the likelihood of developing this complication is even greater. These are significant problems, and at times, they force people to choose therapies that may be less than optimal (e.g., partial, rather than total, cystectomy) for their disease management.

The above problems are amplified in the rare, but tragic, instances of bladder malignancies occurring in children. Tumors are primarily sarcomas and are usually treated with multi-modality therapies—often with organ preservation in mind. Again, information about the outcomes of such treatments is poorly documented, particularly in relation to continued growth, body image, sexual functioning, reproductive capacities, and development of subsequent malignancies. Because of the relative rarity of these tumors, access to a national database is necessary.

Special At-Risk Groups

Research is needed to explain (1) the lower incidence, yet higher mortality, of bladder cancer in women and in African Americans than in white men and (2) the increasing incidence and mortality of bladder cancer with advancing age in both sexes and in all races. With regard to race and ethnicity, Hispanic Americans, who have an incidence of bladder cancer closer to African Americans (i.e., roughly half that of Caucasians), have a mortality rate even lower than that of Caucasians (i.e., roughly half that of African Americans of each sex). The reasons for this are not well understood, but it raises a serious question about whether economics, access to care, and other social factors alone can explain the higher mortalities seen in women, elderly people, and African Americans. Information about other ethnic groups (e.g., Asian Americans and American Indians) is not readily available and is also needed.

Three other groups worth considering for research include

- People with spinal cord injuries, particularly those with long-term indwelling catheters, which place them at higher risk for developing both squamous and transitional cell cancers of the bladder

- Former smokers, who after smoking cessation have a far more rapid decline in their risk for developing lung or esophageal cancer than they do in their risk for developing bladder cancer

- People exposed to industrial and other purported environmental carcinogens

The term urothelial bladder cancer represents a continuum from indolent to aggressive disease. It is of interest to note that although suspected carcinogens predispose for a greater incidence of bladder cancer (except in the young), they do not predispose preferentially for indolent or aggressive cancers—indicating that there is probably a common molecular pathway(s) in the process of urothelial carcinogenesis (cancer development).

Current Research

The Bladder Research Progress Review Group reviewed the bladder research portfolio of the National Institutes of Health (NIH) for February 2001. The review identified a total of 42 individual grants investigating bladder cancer, many of which were components of larger projects. Significantly, only three applications investigate the basic biology of bladder cancer, including such broad areas as tumor invasion, metastases, cell signaling, growth factors and cytokines (hormone-like proteins that regulate the intensity and duration of the immune response), immune system surveillance and detection, angiogenesis, and interactions between the stroma and the urothelium.

Even more important is that none of the grants directly investigate the two most fundamental questions "unique" to bladder cancer: (1) the clonal effect versus the field effect explanation for urothelial cancer's multi-chronotropic behavior (behavior that affects the rate of rhythmic movements in the body) and (2) the degree to which low-grade and high-grade urothelial cancers share common molecular origins and are molecularly separate diseases. Similarly, only two applications investigate one of the most promising and important aspects of bladder cancer research—prevention. None investigated standard or novel epidemiological issues (except as were associated with mechanisms of chemical carcinogenesis), and none could be classified as health services or outcomes research despite overwhelming data indicating the urgent need for these approaches.

Therapeutics is seriously underrepresented also, with only four grants dealing with new approaches, although admittedly the research portfolio provided may have omitted some translational treatment grants.

Research Opportunities

Clearly, research efforts must be refocused in urothelial cancer of the bladder. Most NIH-sponsored research is investigating chemical carcinogenesis, genetics/molecular genetics, and molecular diagnosis. There is a dearth of research on cell signaling, cell regulation, and tumor biology; a great paucity of research on health services; virtually no research on outcomes or on the problems of special groups; virtually no research on behavior and quality-of-life, which is clearly needed; very limited effort on prevention of disease or improving treatment for invasive and metastatic disease; and very little work on developing new ways to image (e.g., virtual endoscopy), diagnose (e.g., contact microscopy), and treat (e.g., genetic therapies) urothelial cancer with methods that may or may not be directly adaptable to other solid tumor sites.

Investigations into the use of technology have only recently begun, and this area is promising because based on the large quantities of tissues and body fluids available and on the predictable nature of this malignancy's behavior, urothelial bladder cancer is a particularly suitable cancer for certain technological approaches such as genomics and proteomics. Much of these research efforts, including participation in clinical trials, would be greatly advanced by developing a suitable infrastructure consisting of multiple centers that would carry out clinical trials and facilitate the obtaining and storing of tissue and fluid samples, along with relevant clinical information and long follow up.

New Technologies

New technologies for facilitating research on urothelial cancer of the bladder include gene therapy, proteomics tools such as immunowalking, and better animal models, including hemizygous, transgenic, and knockout mice.

Gene therapy. Gene therapy is a new and somewhat experimental technology that replaces an absent or faulty gene with a normal, working gene so that the body can manufacture the correct protein or enzyme necessary for cell metabolism and function. Vectors such as viruses are used to carry the normal gene to body cells. The unique accessibility of urothelial tumors, the confined space in which they grow, and, to a large degree, the impermeability of the bladder provide significant opportunities in the area of gene therapy and other targeted therapies.

> **Gene Therapy
> Current Limiting Factors**
>
> - *Inability to deliver constructs to target cells and organs*
>
> - *Inability to assess both targeting and therapeutic gene expression over time*
>
> - *Limitations imposed on the above by development of immune responses to vectors (carriers)*

The ability to deliver vectors locally to the bladder coupled with the ability to repeatedly biopsy the epithelium over time provide a unique platform for assessing these limitations. In addition, the intravesical administration of vectors directly into the bladder where they have direct exposure to target cells, should minimize the vector's exposure to immune system clearance, which is a problem with systemic delivery.

In summary, if these delivery methods are ineffective in the bladder, it is difficult to imagine how they will be successful on the relatively inaccessible sites in which the four more common malignancies (cancer of the prostate, breast, lung, and colon) arise. Similarly, the availability of tissues and fluids, and the current knowledge about bladder cancer's epidemiology, indicate that genomic and proteomic approaches offer great opportunities to define genetic and epigenetic (gene activity rather than in gene structure) alterations in urothelial cells associated with age, gender, race, carcinogen exposure, and exposure avoidance (e.g., smoking and smoking cessation). These studies are likely to provide critical insights into the puzzling epidemiologic and demographic observations discussed previously. This information will ultimately result in improved disease detection, prevention, and possibly treatment.

Immunowalking and proteomics. Immunowalking is a variant of proteomics, the study of protein expression by the genes. Immunowalking has enormous potential for facilitating research on the processes of malignant urothelial transformation and progression. The approach makes use of proteomic technologies to reveal and identify proteins that are differentially expressed in fresh tumors and normal epithelium. Thereafter, specific antibodies against the differentially expressed proteins are used (immunowalking) to stain serial cryostat sections of specimens obtained from tumor-bearing patients who have undergone removal of malignant bladder tissue. The urothelium of these patients is expected to exhibit a spectrum of abnormalities, ranging from early stages of transformation to invasive disease.

Better animal models. Classical animal models for bladder cancer studies include carcinogen-induced models in rats, dogs, and mice. Cancer is induced in these animals after intravesical or oral administration of carcinogens. A limitation of these models is that the types of cancers that develop frequently include significant amounts of squamous cell carcinoma rather than transitional cell carcinoma, which is the far more common bladder cancer histology in humans.

Furthermore, these classical animal models do not typically result in metastatic disease because the animals' lives are limited by obstruction of the ureters and kidney failure. Although this may be the normal course of untreated human bladder cancer, the models do not address the major cause of bladder cancer death in humans today—uncontrollable metastatic disease.

Even with the above-mentioned drawbacks, these classical models have contributed significantly to our understanding of bladder carcinogenesis and the development of immunotherapy involving the intravesical administration of bacillus Calmette-Guerin (BCG), a bacterium used as what is thought to be a non-specific immune system stimulant. BCG is dissolved in normal saline solution and administered into the bladder, where it binds to the bladder tissue and stimulates an immune response that interferes with the growth of local tumors. Classical animal models have also contributed to the development of new chemoprevention agents, currently under phase III testing.

A more recent study of p53 hemizygous mice that had a normal lifespan and had not developed cancer may be very useful for chemoprevention studies. P53, a protein that normally suppresses tumors, actually causes them when it is mutated. In the hemizygous mouse, only one normal p53 allele is inherited from parents, the other allele is missing. By feeding a mutagenic substance excreted in urine, urothelial cells are exposed to this chemical, and mutation of the remaining p53 allele results in a defective gene product. Thus, it is not surprising that bladder cancers can be induced in the mice by feeding them with p-cresidine, an azo dye analogue that is carcinogenic. The p53 hemizygous mice developed cancers within four to six months with this regimen, while wild-type littermates required nine to twelve months to develop cancer (because the mutagen had to mutate both copies of p53 in the same target cell).

Xenograft mouse models of bladder cancer have also been useful in research. A xenograft is a graft transferred from an animal of one species to an animal of another species. These mice receive human bladder tumor cells that are injected either intravenously or intraperitoneally into organs other than the bladder. Tumors often "take" because the host mouse is immunodeficient, so it does not reject the cells from a foreign species as an immunologically intact animal would. Importantly, as one study showed, the organ environment provides important and specific signals in tumor development. In another study, a xenograft model with bladder cancer was developed to study metastasis and therapies. More recently, tumor cells were generated that express green fluorescent proteins that emit light when stimulated. Tumors developing from such cells in the bladder can be monitored for metastasis and measured non-invasively using a specific light source.

Transgenics is a relatively new technique that uses genetically modified mice to drive bladder cancer development. The uroplakin-II gene's promoter, which is only expressed in urothelium, has been used to drive the expression of a viral protein, "large T antigen," that results in both superficial and invasive bladder cancers. More recently, the uroplakin promoter has been used to drive urothelial over-expression of the RAS oncogene, resulting in mice with only superficial papillary cancers. Another study found that the FABP gene's promoter can also drive tissue-specific gene expression in epithelium. In addition, these promoters potentially could be used to develop other transgenic bladder cancer models.

Because genetically modified animals are a powerful resource in studying the role of putative oncogenes (genes that may foster malignancies if mutated or activated) and suppressor genes in the carcinogenic process, additional transgenic and knockout animals should be derived. Transgenic animals have had new DNA introduced into their germ cells through injection into an ovum. Knockout animals are genetically engineered animals whose genome has been altered by recombination so that a gene is deleted. These animals would also be important for studies of growth factors, cellular interactions, and, possibly, immunity in both normal and pathologic processes.

Several promoters, such as those of various keratins, frequently have been used to drive gene expression in urothelial tissues such as the skin. The urothelium expresses these keratins as well, although at lower levels. Thus, such transgenics may also have bladder abnormalities. This phenomenon is not well appreciated, and the bladder is often not even examined for phenotypic changes when keratin-specific transgenic and knockout

mice are studied. Other transgenic animals may also show unexpected bladder phenotypes that are not identified or explored because the bladder is frequently not included in the tissues evaluated.

Finally, because some genes are essential for development, some knockout mice do not reach adulthood. Similarly, because bladder cancer is associated with aging, altered gene expression may not be a lifelong phenomenon. Therefore, it has been recommended that inducible systems should have a number of applications for examining gene function at selected times in postnatal life, under selected physiologic or pathophysiologic conditions.

Providing investigators with readily accessible information about these models is as important as developing them. A Genetically Altered Animal Models Database of Bladder Cancer, similar to one developed by the National Heart, Lung, and Blood Institute (http://www.nhlbi.nih.gov/resources/medres/transgen.htm), would provide information on useful animal models and prevent wasteful duplication of effort. This is another example of the infrastructural support that is needed to promote bladder cancer research.

Bladder Cancer as a Model System for Research

The bladder is an ideal model organ system. In that capacity, bladder cancer could be used as a model to study

- **New technological developments relevant to other tumor sites that are less accessible for study**—The delivery of chemicals directly into the bladder has been done for years in the form of intravesical therapy. However, the delivery of new agents (e.g., vectors for genetic manipulations, vaccines, labeled agents for photodynamic diagnostic tests, and new treatments) is already being explored, but far less so than would be expected considering this disease's anatomic location.

- **Tumor-host (immune) interaction**—The natural history and current therapy of human bladder cancer provide outstanding opportunities for dissecting immune mechanisms in the bladder, including those related to tumors. Malignant tissue is readily and repeatedly accessible, and tumor-associated immune populations and cytokines (proteins that regulate the intensity and duration of the immune response and mediate cell-cell communication) could be sampled via routinely scheduled cystoscopy and biopsy (standard of care), bladder washings, or the collection of fluids or cells and molecules normally shed in urine. With these specimens, the tumor-host interaction could be examined over time. In addition, the routine use of intravesical BCG for the treatment of superficial bladder cancer could provide a surrogate antigen (target) that would allow investigators to study the induction and effector arms of the immune response and to investigate the tumor's effects on immune function.

New Prevention Strategies

Clearly, the best way to reduce bladder cancer mortality is to prevent its development. Proposed strategies include avoidance of putative carcinogen exposure (e.g., smoking) and reduction of carcinogen exposure (e.g., increased fluid ingestion to dilute carcinogens). These strategies appear attractive, although their success has not been tested in a prospective fashion. In the case of rare specific exposures, including exposure to *A. franghi* in Chinese weight-loss herbs and to arsenic-related substances in contaminated well water, regulatory measures have proven quite effective in lowering urothelial cancer incidence, although effects on disease-specific mortality have yet to be reported.

A complementary approach to avoidance has been the use of chemopreventive agents. Several agents have prevented carcinogen-induced bladder tumors in preclinical animal studies. In clinical prevention trials, some of these agents appear promising in other human tumor sites. Currently in phase III testing in the United States are the oral polyamine synthesis inhibitor, DFMO; the cyclooxygenase 2 (COX 2) inhibitor, celocoxib; and the vitamin A analog, 4HPF. Results of these trials are not yet available. In prior phase III trials, other retinoids—vitamin B6 and alpha tocopherol (a vitamin E analog)—have had mixed or negative results, and some retinoids have been quite toxic.

Most of these agents have been, or are being, tested in secondary preventive settings on patients whose superficial tumors were completely resected but who are at risk for developing recurrences. Although this represents an attractive and large population to study, depending on trial design, this may be testing both prevention of new tumors and treatment of existing ones. However, without success at the secondary level, it would be hard to justify a primary preventative trial specifically for bladder cancer because of the much greater sample sizes required. A presumed assumption in the design of some of the secondary trials is that preventing low-grade tumors may also be helpful in preventing high-grade ones. Although data exist to the contrary, most of the clinical, epidemiological, and molecular evidence appears to support this hypothesis.

Promising natural products include plant estrogens (phytoestrogens) such as genestine, which can inhibit growth factor tyrosine kinases, should also be tested. However, significant further effort must be placed in this area. Along with new candidate agents, perhaps the greatest need in prevention studies is that of characterizing intermediate molecular marker endpoints of premalignancy, the reversal of which correlate with a successful outcome. Finally, a combination of agents, including a combination with existing intravesical therapies, is beginning to be pursued and is theoretically attractive.

New Molecular Markers

Compared with many other tumor sites, much progress has been made in the molecular diagnosis of urothelial cancers. Several molecular epigenetic and genetic markers have the capacity to diagnose 80 percent to 95 percent of Grade 3 tumors and 40 percent to 80 percent of low-grade ones. These tests have generated considerable financial interest, with an eye on ultimately replacing more invasive means of diagnosis and monitoring, particularly cystoscopy.

To date, no commercially available test has the sensitivity, particularly for low-grade tumors, to be useful by itself in establishing an initial diagnosis or in monitoring patients. However, several markers in various stages of testing and commercial development have this potential.

The most promising new molecular markers include Immunocyt, a combination of three monoclonal antibodies to bladder-cancer-associated antigens and cytology; hyaluronidase and hyaluronic acid; BLCA-4, a nuclear matrix protein; Survivan, a protein that inhibits programmed cell death (apoptosis); telomerase activity and protein; several tests of genetic instability in DNA in urine using a panel of marker DNA microsatellites (compared with genomic DNA); and fluorescence *in situ* hybridization (FISH) analysis of a combination of chromosomal markers.

Although aggressive attempts to define a market for these products continue, it is possible that some combination of markers could be scored in such a way that would make them have sufficient sensitivity and acceptable specificity to be able to replace cystoscopy in diagnosis and monitoring. Eventually these markers could be used for screening demographically defined, at-risk populations (e.g., middle-aged and elderly male smokers and former smokers) in a non-invasive or minimally invasive fashion.

Such combination studies are desperately needed, but industry has a limited interest in these trials because a commercial competitor may benefit more than the sponsoring company. This problem also occurs with innovative use of combinations of agents in preventive and therapeutic strategies. Additionally, detection and particularly screening endeavors are ideally suited for mathematical modeling to optimize and streamline study designs and strategies before extensive clinical testing occurs. For example, repetitive reagent strip testing for blood in the urine (hematuria) has been shown to have sufficient sensitivity for screening purposes; however, the specificity of this reagent strip could be improved with a second tier of marker tests that would determine which person with hematuria should proceed to cystoscopy. This strategy would be more attractive to potential screening subjects, but it awaits the combination marker analysis and appropriate modeling.

Once a combination of markers is available, a phase III, randomized, prospective, controlled trial of bladder cancer screening is clearly warranted by the

- High incidence of the disease

- Great success in treating superficial tumors with a relatively non-morbid means

- Serious deficiencies in treating more locally advanced and metastatic cancers with means that are highly morbid

- Compelling clinical evidence that virtually all people who die of urothelial cancer (those with metastases) have malignancies that invade the bladder muscle at the time that metastases occur or before

> ## Promising Molecular Markers
>
> - *Immunocyt*
>
> - *Hyaluronidase and hyaluronic acid*
>
> - *BLCA-4*
>
> - *Survivan*
>
> - *Telomerase activity and protein*
>
> - *Fluorescence in situ hybridization (FISH) analysis*
>
> - *Tests of genetic instability in DNA in urine using a panel of marker DNA microsatellites*

Because between 70 percent and 90 percent of all people with muscle-invading bladder cancer currently have that level of invasion at the time of their initial bladder cancer diagnosis (i.e., they do not come from the enormous pool of people with previously treated superficial tumors), the need for earlier detection as a major means of reducing bladder cancer mortality is obvious.

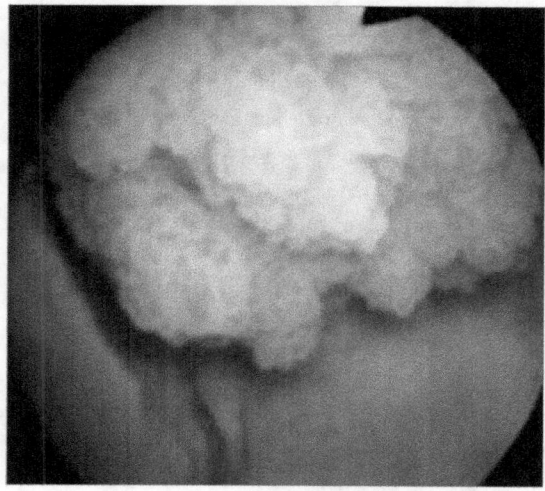

A cystoscopic image of a superficial papillary tumor of the bladder. *(Photo Credit: Healthcommunities.com, Inc., Bladder Cancer on urologychannel.* All rights reserved. http://www.urologychannel.com. Copyright 2002. Healthcommunities.com, Inc.)*

Requirements for Bladder Cancer Research

Although it could be argued that important initiatives and funding mechanisms for novel approaches to bladder cancer are lacking, only 50 percent of all NIH-funded research in bladder cancer is occurring through traditional, investigator-initiated (i.e., RO1, R21/29, and PO1 grants that are entirely on bladder cancer) mechanisms. This indicates that more creative requests for applications (RFAs) and other funding mechanisms are not necessarily the only answer. Alternatively, prostate cancer and breast cancer have recruited major investigators from other fields because of the funds available, and this lesson could well be applied to bladder cancer, which, although it is the fifth

most common non-cutaneous malignancy in the United States, lags well behind these diseases in overall funding.

If even a small but proportionate increase is made for bladder cancer research (a justified increase based on the disease's incidence), it is likely that huge strides could be made, if in no other area than in equalizing mortalities in women, elderly people, and African Americans to the mortalities of middle-aged Caucasian men. This alone would cut bladder mortality by 20 percent.

If the economical use of public funds to address health care concerns is truly the highest priority, the magnitude of support going to bladder cancer research seems disproportionately low when compared with support for research on other malignancies and diseases. This is particularly true because so much is known about bladder cancer and because it is likely that relatively simple interventions such as earlier detection, smoking cessation (with a particular emphasis on people at risk for, or who already have, bladder cancer), and education (directed particularly at demographic groups with disproportionately high morbidity and mortality) might have a major beneficial impact in reducing mortality and morbidity.

Tissue and Specimen Banks

Some of the most exciting and novel scientific approaches such as informatics, proteomics, genomics, and novel imaging—approaches that are particularly suitable for bladder cancer applications—have significantly lagged behind efforts in other tumor sites. Admittedly, in creating useful tissue banks and arrays, technical challenges arise in harvesting, dissecting, and orienting bladder tumor tissue. However, with care, these and other technical problems can be surmounted to obtain appropriate specimens for array preparation and banking. This often requires an interested team of investigators and infrastructural support.

Advances in cancer are tightly linked to the availability of tissue specimens for study. Tissue is a snapshot picture of a tumor, but a complete biology is linked to that tissue becoming malignant. Molecular changes that would be reflected in outcome are already present in the tumor tissue when it is resected. Adequate access to tumor and normal tissue is a chronic problem for research in cancer. In the bladder, the cancer process is a continuum from normal cells to abnormal tissue development (dysplasia) to localized tumors to invasive and metastatic disease, with both flat and papillary (exophytic and endophytic) pre-malignant and pre-invasive stages. To facilitate research in bladder cancer, the development of an extensive network of tissue banks, both institution-based and cooperative, is essential.

Tissue and specimen banks will require significant support for storage, registration, and dissemination of the tissue. Tissue banks will need to include frozen specimens (in liquid nitrogen) as well as paraffin-embedded tissue. Ideally, tissue and specimen banks should contain simultaneously obtained, ostensibly normal, epithelium from the same patient's bladder. Moreover, these specimen samples must be tied to complete clinical, epidemiologic, demographic, genetic, and other information, with accurate and long-term follow up.

Tumor Registry Systems

Tissue and specimen banks are also integral parts of tumor registry systems that record outcomes. These registries will be of great importance in the development of better prognostic markers, which requires sufficient tissue correlated with known outcomes.

Currently, the number, size, and quality of such banks of malignant and normal tissues and exfoliated cells (with good clinical correlation and follow-up) are inadequate for the needs of modern molecular research in bladder cancer, and there is no access to samples (and clinical information) for worthy investigators

outside laboratories where such banks reside. Establishment of these banks, with a ready distribution of high-quality specimens, would greatly facilitate research.

High Throughput Methodologies

High throughput technologies are capable of performing a large number of tests in a short period of time. A number of new high throughput technologies have been recently developed that will dramatically alter bladder cancer research. Laser capture microdissection (LCM) allows the collection of small, pure populations of cells. The current emphasis of research in the post-genome era is the profiling of cDNA expression (using DNA chips) and its correlation with protein expression (using both immunologic and mass-spectroscopic identification of proteins). Now tissue arrays with samples of hundreds of tumors are available.

This high throughput technology moves the study of cancer from in-depth observations on a few specimens to the study and verification of observations on a sufficient number of cancers, reaching statistically valid conclusions in very brief periods of time. Some of these techniques are applicable to urine specimens (both soluble and cellular components) as well. High throughput methodologies offer the opportunity to define proteins that would be useful in making diagnoses, formulating prognoses, and monitoring patients.

Bioinformatics Systems

A far bigger hurdle to overcome, and one that is by no means unique to bladder cancer research, is the enormous barrier to developing tissue and specimen banks with critically important clinical, correlative, and follow-up information that is placed by institutional review boards. These constraints are based on concerns about patient confidentiality, informed consent, potential financial profit, patient reimbursement, and other ethical issues. A national policy, spearheaded by the National Institutes of Health and the National Academy of Sciences, but accepted by the public and other constituencies, is needed immediately to overcome these hurdles.

Both the development of strong inter-institutional tissue banks with correlative clinical information and the use of high throughput methodologies for the analysis of tumors require the development of bioinformatics systems. Such systems will benefit all disciplines that use tissue and that are engaged in high throughput methodologies. The funding needs for such resources exceed what has traditionally been available through normal granting mechanisms. Additional financial support will be required to make sure that data are collected and disseminated.

Review Groups with Knowledge of Urothelial Cancer

Clearly, bladder cancer research is relatively underfunded, but it might also be under applied for. Data were not available to the authors of this report on the number of research applications accepted or rejected for urothelial cancer as opposed to other cancers. However, review groups with a particular interest in, and knowledge of, this disease might greatly improve the prospects for funding—particularly of R01 and R29 grants.

Grants are often sent to more general study sections (no data were provided on this) where reviewers unfamiliar with the nuances of bladder cancer may not be able to fairly appraise the specific merits of an application in terms of this unique disease site. In such review groups, lack of appreciation of models and approaches that have specific relevance to bladder cancer (e.g., carcinogenic models and use of endoscopic evaluations) but are not directly applicable to tumors with which the reviewers may be more familiar mitigates against the success of a bladder cancer application in the peer-review process.

Epidemiology and Basic Scientific Mechanisms of Disease Research

More research on epidemiology and basic biological mechanisms of urothelial cancer is clearly needed.

Multi-Center Programs and Networks

Mechanisms for funding multi-center programs with sufficient infrastructure support to promote novel investigations (and indeed an emphasis on this) and recruitment of new investigators may be productive ways to sponsor further research. Recently a Bladder Cancer Special Program of Research Excellence (SPORE) was awarded to MD Anderson Tumor Institute in Houston, Texas; this may indicate that there is an awareness of this problem.

Public Interest and Educational Efforts

These efforts are clearly important, and they have been enormously effective for prostate cancer and breast cancer research. Patient advocacy groups also do not exist for cancer of the bladder as they do for many other malignant and non-malignant diseases. Such groups not only improve research and educational efforts, but also permit clinical researchers to be more aware of the needs and priorities of patients.

Hubert Humphrey

Bladder Cancer

In 1967, Hubert Humphrey, Vice President of the United States and a presidential candidate, discovered blood in his urine—often the first sign of urinary tract disease. The vice president immediately consulted his doctors, who examined his bladder with a cystoscope, but found nothing that appeared abnormal. His physicians also sent samples of his urine and bladder tissue to pathologists who performed tests for abnormal cells, but none of the samples positively established that cancer was present. A tissue sample from a tiny spot in Humphrey's bladder did show irregularities in some cells; however pathologists were unable to agree on a diagnosis.

Although it was somewhat controversial, Humphrey's physicians decided on a period of watchful waiting. The vice president continued his campaign for the presidency, but lost the election to Richard Nixon, who ironically declared a "War on Cancer" in 1972. Six years later, Humphrey lost his personal war on cancer.

Vice President Humphrey's medical history reveals much about the difficulty of diagnosing bladder cancer. Technology available at the time was unable to detect cancer cells until 1969, two years after his symptoms first appeared. Biopsies taken of tumors at that time revealed "*in situ* cancer," that is, localized malignant tumors in the epithelium, the mucous tissue lining the inner surface of the bladder. By 1973, a biopsy report noted "pre-invasive malignancy," cancer that was about to invade underlying tissue and muscle. Although Humphrey received radiation therapy and localized chemotherapy for the disease, by 1976 the cancer had become invasive, necessitating removal of the bladder. Lymph nodes removed during surgery indicated that the cancer had spread to other parts of his body. Hubert Humphrey died of cancer in January 1978 at the age of 66.

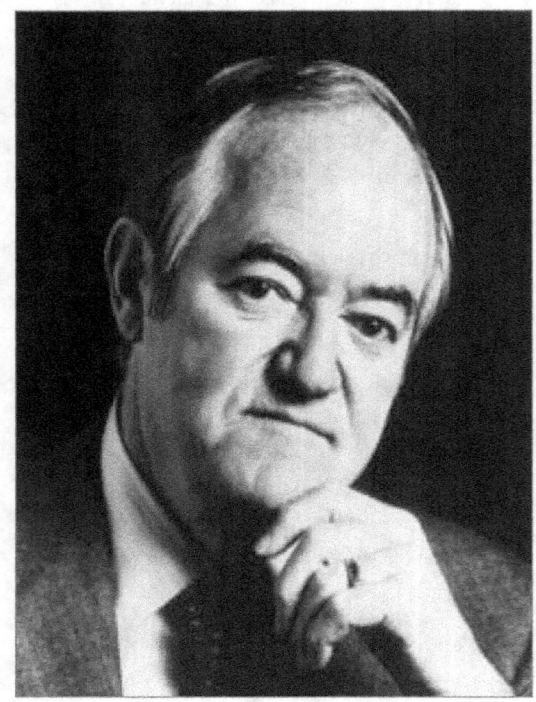

(Photo Credit: U.S. Senate Historical Office)

Bladder cancer is frequently undetected in its early stages, even today. It usually does not cause symptoms such as blood in the urine or frequent urinations until large tumors are present. Even when symptoms do appear in early stages, finding cancerous cells among thousands of normal cells in urine or in biopsied bladder tissue is difficult and often impossible. Clearly, development of markers that point to early disease could reduce the high morbidity and mortality associated with bladder cancer.

Better tests appear to be on the horizon. In the past decade, advances in biotechnologies and the science of genomics and proteomics have laid the groundwork for early diagnosis. New technologies allow for replication of DNA samples from scarce genes, and new types of DNA analysis are now capable of detecting cells with genetic mutations.

One preliminary screening tool for bladder cancer in its early stages was tested in 1994 by a team of researchers at Johns Hopkins University School of Medicine, using Humphrey's urine and tissue samples. The team obtained permission from Humphrey's widow to use a urine sample collected in 1967 and a tumor sample collected several years later. Armed with new knowledge about mutations in genes and a new technique, the polymerase chain reaction (PCR), which allows scientists to make multiple copies of DNA from scarce genes, the researchers set out to see if cells sloughed off into Humphrey's urine would show signs of disease.

In studying the cells of the tumor sample (collected in 1973 when cancer was visible in Humphrey's bladder), researchers discovered that the cells had mutations in the p53 gene. Certain mutations in this gene are now recognized as the cause of 60 percent of very aggressive bladder cancers. In Humphrey's case, one DNA building block, adenine, had replaced another, thymine, in the sequence. The mutation was not present in the non-cancerous tissues of Humphrey's bladder.

In a separate, but similar procedure, researchers took the urine sample collected when Humphrey was first examined in 1967 and again used PCR. They discovered that even when physicians could not determine whether cancer was present, cells in Humphrey's urine had markers of the type of mutation that caused his cancer.

Although researchers have demonstrated how a marker for incipient disease could lead to early diagnosis and treatment, developing a test that has the sensitivity to detect all types of bladder cancer is not so simple. Microsatellite analysis has been available for approximately 10 years, but it is still not a standard tool or test. Mutations in p53 are not present in all bladder cancers, and in fact, many different mutations in this gene can cause the disease, which is strongly associated with environmental toxins and smoking.

According to the American Cancer Society, the incidence of bladder cancer in the United States increased 30 percent between 1985 and 2000. Currently, between 250,000 and 500,000 people have this disease. Many are elderly men and women who face years of treatment that includes surgical removal of the bladder, urinary diversion, high-dose pelvic radiotherapy, and multi-drug chemotherapy, treatments that are not only expensive, but also highly morbid. With better preventive strategies and more sensitive molecular screening tools that take advantage of the great strides made in genomics and proteomics, the pain and suffering caused by bladder cancer could be reduced.

SECTION C METHODOLOGIES & TECHNOLOGIES FOR FUTURE RESEARCH

Bladder research would benefit from recent advances in biotechnology that have created rapid progress in other areas of scientific endeavor. All areas of bladder research and all patients with bladder-associated health problems would specifically benefit from the following advances:

- New biologic (cellular or molecular) and functional imaging techniques and genomics and proteomics techniques to identify persons at risk for bladder disease or dysfunction

- Bioengineering technology such as stem cells, gene therapy, and tissue engineering techniques that allow repair, replacement, or even prevention of abnormal bladder tissue or function

As rapidly as research has progressed in proteomics and genomics, pharmacologic discovery aimed at modulating, augmenting, or blocking specific receptors has also progressed. New drug delivery systems allowing drug delivery at a specific time and place are possible, and the bladder is an ideal organ in which to deliver them.

Methodologies such as bioinformatics and epidemiology and advances in computer technology permit linkage of patient and disease data and allow clinical research to be performed using databases that surpass previous capabilities and capacities. The methodologies and technologies apply new rigor to clinical trials involving outcomes evaluations and neural networks. In studies of complex conditions, bioinformatics and biostatistics allow scientists to make inferences and conclusions that were previously impossible to make.

At this time in medicine, clinical research is severely challenged. Clinical investigators have less time for clinical research because of the increasing complexities involved in performing their day-to-day patient care activities. Clinical trials are poorly funded. Clinical research is expensive, and human research is highly regulated requiring high degrees of organization and support. Many bladder diseases have a long natural history, and outcomes trials must be undertaken over many years, facts that make clinical research even more complicated.

CHAPTER 13

CLINICAL TRIALS IN LOWER URINARY TRACT RESEARCH

Methodologies & Technologies for Future Research

DID YOU KNOW?

→ Few clinical studies have been conducted on disease of the lower urinary tract.

→ Enormous opportunities are currently available for data gathering and examining best practices in bladder disease management.

Summary and Recommendations

Clinical trials related to bladder disease are scarce. Currently, the National Institute of Diabetes and Digestive and Kidney Diseases (NIDDK) of the National Institutes of Health (NIH) is conducting clinical trials or programs in only four areas of bladder disease—bladder cancer, interstitial cystitis, incontinence, and obstruction.

Enormous opportunities for data gathering and for examination of best practices and management of bladder disease exist through clinical trials, yet they have been under utilized and under funded in the area of bladder research. Examination of issues that have been impediments might provide an incentive to programs applying for future clinical trials in bladder research.

The Bladder Research Progress Review Group prioritized the research opportunities and implementation recommendations for clinical trials activities. Their recommendations are as follows:

First Priority

⇨ **Fund pilot studies with high-risk, high-gain potential**

⇨ **Prioritize clinical studies lacking short-term gain in which funding from other sources is unlikely, such as**

- Alternative therapies (e.g., saw palmetto)

- Prevention studies (e.g., childbirth injuries)

- Long-term outcome studies

- Behavioral studies

- Long-term management and surgical trials

➡ Develop a core clinical trial resource center (NIDDK) with core consultation services in

- Biostatistics

- Epidemiology

- Outcomes evaluation

- Ethics

Second Priority

➡ Encourage establishment of multi-center studies to examine low-incidence and high-impact bladder diseases or problems

➡ Provide industrial partnering grants to piggyback basic or epidemiologic research (e.g., examination of potential molecular markers for detection, monitoring, and screening)

Current Research and Opportunities for Research

A number of initiatives would benefit many investigators and offer advances in understanding diseases that have few treatment options. These initiatives would

- Standardize tissue and specimen banking issues, particularly relating to prioritization of studies and ethical issues

- Provide infrastructure expertise and support perhaps at regional or national centers for biostatistical, epidemiologic, ethical, and outcomes clinical research

- Provide specific support for pilot clinical trials that lack corporate interest or support, such as high-risk but high-gain treatment of specific complex or severe bladder problems.

Some areas in which clinical trials may offer advances include diabetes, development, cancer, incontinence, infection, inflammation, and obstruction.

Diabetes

Although the NIH has an organized infrastructure of research programs in diabetes, none of these programs appears to be currently conducting research related to the lower urinary tract. Better communication among ongoing studies in the diabetes program may allow identification of studies related to diabetic bladder and its risk factors. An examination of the epidemiology and risk factors for bladder involvement in diabetes is needed, and this could be done within the existing infrastructure as listed below:

- Mouse Models of Diabetic Complications Consortium

- Therapeutic Approaches to Diabetes Mellitus Program

- Type 1 Diabetes Clinical Trials Program

- Type 2 Diabetes Clinical Trials Program

- Diabetes Prevention Program

- Endocrine Pancreas Program

- Complications Genetics Program

- Type 1 Diabetes Epidemiology Research Program

- Type 2 Diabetes Epidemiology Research Program

- National Diabetes Data Group

- Diabetes Mellitus Interagency Coordinating Committee

- National Diabetes Education Program

- Diabetes Centers Program

Development

The NIH should conduct longitudinal behavioral studies of voiding patterns and of subjects' elimination history to track the natural history of voiding problems from childhood to adult. (e.g.. 30-year studies)

Cancer

The NIH should conduct the following research studies on cancer of the lower urinary tract:

- Advanced cancer and outcomes

- Assessment of patient populations for risk

- Use of the bladder as a biologic model for development and delivery of various therapeutic interventions such as gene therapy

- Potential of supplemental studies related to cancer biology to be added to cancer trials

Incontinence

The NIH should provide support for

- Small Business Innovation Research (SBIR) grants and joint venture research with the pharmaceutical companies

- Biofeedback and Kegel exercises for voiding dysfunction

Infection and Inflammation

The NIH should conduct studies that examine and evaluate

- Longitudinal follow-up of the natural history of interstitial cystitis

- Treatments and emergence of antimicrobial resistance

- Significance of bacteriuria in the neurogenic and catheterized bladder

- Natural history of bladder function in persons with recurrent urinary tract infections

- Risk for bacterial and fungal urinary tract infection

Obstruction

The NIH should investigate the following:

- Treatment of benign prostatic hyperplasia (BPH) using alternative therapies such as antioxidants

- Bladder and ureteral obstruction and their effects on muscle, upper urinary tract, and kidney function. with examination for markers of renal failure (longitudinal study)

CHAPTER 14

EPIDEMIOLOGY OF BLADDER DISORDERS

Methodologies & Technologies for Future Research

DID YOU KNOW?

→ Lack of data on risk factors in urethral and bladder dysfunction limits therapeutic and preventive efforts.

→ Lack of information on prevalence and incidence of lower urinary tract dysfunction prevents accurate estimates of health care costs and resource planning.

Summary and Recommendations

Prevalence, incidence, natural history of, and risk factors for urethral and bladder dysfunction are essential core research areas. However, the National Institute of Diabetes and Digestive and Kidney Diseases (NIDDK) has traditionally funded few epidemiologic research projects. In 2001, for example, the NIDDK Epidemiologic Research Portfolio was only funded at $5.3 million. This is in sharp contrast to funding for basic science ($41.7 million), clinical trials ($8.3 million), and applied and developmental research ($8.8 million).

Data on the prevalence and incidence of disease are important because they are used to assess the burden of disease. This information is vitally important to estimate health care costs and to direct resource planning. Identification of risk factors provides the foundation for determining what causes a disease and how to prevent it. Our current paucity of information on established risk factors in urethral and bladder dysfunction limits preventive efforts and highlights the need for increased epidemiologic research funding.

The Bladder Research Progress Review Group made the following recommendations for future research efforts:

▣ **Increase markedly the number and funding of epidemiology research— particularly longitudinal studies—to estimate incidence and to determine the natural history of the disease. These studies should**

- Use validated and standardized questionnaires in epidemiological studies. (Most epidemiologic studies in the past ascertained outcomes by patient self-report. Ideally, self-report measures should be validated and standardized.)

- Obtain representative samples of target populations and well-conducted data collections for epidemiologic studies.

- Use cross-sectional studies as efficient and reasonable methods to determine prevalence and to identify potential risk factors.

- Provide careful measurement of a wide variety of potential risk factors and a very large sample to allow for statistical adjustment for multiple potential-confounding variables and careful follow-up over several years (longitudinal studies).

- Study risk factors to define causality.

- Append ancillary studies of urethra and bladder dysfunction to large ongoing longitudinal studies for an efficient means to evaluate incidence and natural history of disease.

▣ Conduct economic analyses to assist with more rational, effective, and economically sound medical decision-making.

Background

During the past three decades, rapidly increasing health care costs have outpaced inflation and consumed more than 13 percent of the United States gross domestic product according to the Economic Report of the President. Cost-effectiveness analyses incorporate data on both health outcomes and costs and comprehensively describe the relative value of alternative interventions for a specific medical condition. Few data exist on the cost-of-illness or cost-effectiveness of treatments for urethral and bladder dysfunction. In addition, no data are available on patient preference (utility) for treatment and health outcomes. For economic analyses in each area of urethral and bladder disease, measurement of direct and indirect costs, patient preferences (utilities) and economic evaluation, preferably cost-effectiveness analysis, are needed in future studies.

Research Requirements and Impediments

Requirements

The Bladder Research Progress Review Group has identified critical needs for epidemiologic research in the areas of workforce issues, infrastructure, tissue and specimen banks, and interactions with biotechnology and pharmaceutical companies.

Workforce. The area of bladder dysfunction research has few well-trained clinical researchers. A complete funding program for development of a cadre of well-trained clinical investigators would include funding for fellows, young faculty, and mid-level faculty.

Support for two- to three-year fellowship training programs in clinical research methods is essential. To be successful, fellows require focused didactic training, expert mentoring, and a clear research plan. Because urology and urogynecology are surgical specialties, a 20 percent to 25 percent clinical activities restriction should be reconsidered. A possible reasonable clinical activity level would be limited to 25 percent for the first year, 50 percent for the second year, and 50 percent for the third year.

At the early investigator level, four- to five-year funding after fellowship (similar to the Women's Reproductive Health Research Career Development Award of the National Institute of Child and Human Development, which is modeled after a K23 award) is necessary to allow for professional development. At the mid-career level, funding (K24 award) for four to five years is needed for mid-level faculty to mentor fellows and junior faculty.

Infrastructure. Currently, the basic mechanisms of urethral and bladder dysfunction remain largely speculative; data on prevalence, incidence, and associated risk factors are limited; major gaps exist in our knowledge of therapeutic efficacy; and information about the economic impact of urethral and bladder dysfunction is scarce. Multi-disciplinary, multi-center research programs with representation from departments of obstetrics, gynecology, and reproductive sciences, urology, epidemiology, and biostatistics, geriatrics, and medicine are necessary to foster and facilitate research in clinical and basic science of the lower urinary tract.

Funding mechanisms are needed to establish the infrastructure necessary to support the model of a "bench-to-bedside" collaborative research paradigm and to allow direct translation of scientific data to improved patient care. In collaboration with basic scientists, clinical epidemiologists can answer interesting and novel scientific questions.

Tissue and specimen banks. Tissue, blood, or urine samples could be collected and banked in well-characterized cohorts.

Interactions with pharmaceutical and biotechnological companies. Industry-sponsored research is an engine of progress and opportunities. Most clinical trials of new drugs and devices are sponsored by industry. These clinical trials are an important part of the foundation of clinical practice and public health, and they can be a source of important advances in medical science.

Industry sponsorship generates pressures to produce research results and reports that may be favorable to the marketing of drugs and devices. Academic investigators can increase the objectivity and quality of this research by assuming leadership roles in study design and by conducting research and disseminating results. This engagement can lead not only to more appropriate use of treatments and tests, but also opportunities for generating and testing new scientific ideas.

Impediments

Historically, the vast majority of research supported by the NIDDK has been in basic science. Most reviewers and consultants are senior basic science investigators who are not trained in clinical research methodology and design. Study sections and planning meetings for future research agendas should consider including senior epidemiologists from other fields who are familiar with the importance and quality of epidemiologic research.

Research Opportunities

Effective prevention requires an understanding of the causes and natural history of diseases of the urethra and bladder. The BRPRG recommends that research

➡ **Markedly increase the number and funding of epidemiology research and specifically longitudinal studies that will:**

- Determine the prevalence and incidence of, and risk factors associated with, urethral and bladder dysfunction, especially those that are preventable or modifiable

- Establish the burden of these dysfunctions in economic, health, and quality of life terms

- Test the effectiveness of risk factor modification to prevent or decrease severity of disease

➡ **Support training of fellows, junior faculty, and mentors in epidemiologic research**

➡ **Establish review and funding mechanisms that will support the infrastructure to build multi-disciplinary clinical and basic science research**

CHAPTER 15

EMERGING TECHNOLOGIES AND PHARMACOLOGY

Methodologies & Technologies for Future Research

DID YOU KNOW?

→ Current bladder reconstruction techniques use tissue from a person's GI tract that can cause significant complications, including infection and cancer.

→ Bulking agents used in current procedures to relieve both severe urinary incontinence and urinary reflux are not entirely biocompatible.

→ Stem cell populations associated with the urinary tract have been identified.

→ Development and applications of tissue bioengineering techniques could enable people to "self-donate" an organ such as a bladder.

An estimated 35 million Americans suffer from bladder disease, and most of them have problems that are chronic. Dysfunction of the lower urinary tract can be the result of congenital problems, inflammation, infection, or various lesions of the nervous system. These diseases and conditions interfere with the bladder's ability to function as a low-pressure storage and emptying vehicle. The outcome is both reduced bladder elasticity and urinary incontinence, with subsequent deterioration of the upper urinary tract. Bladder disease often involves or results in the loss of tissue structure or function, problems that lead to increased morbidity and poor quality of life.

In the future, emerging technologies such as tissue engineering, stem cells, and genomics will play an important role in the diagnosis and treatment of bladder disease. After an extensive review of past and current research on the lower urinary tract, the Bladder Research Progress Review Group (BRPRG) made the following recommendations for future research on these technologies:

➔ **Conduct stem cell therapy and tissue engineering research of the bladder, urethra, and pelvic floor, with the goals of**

- Increased understanding of cell and developmental biology

- Development of cell therapy

- Development of tissue and organ replacement

➔ **Develop instrumentation for minimally invasive diagnosis of lower urinary tract disorders. Instrumentation should include**

- Functional imaging

- Urodynamics

- Biomechanical assessment

➡ **Establish the appropriate infrastructure, training, and core facilities for research, including**

- Genomics and proteomics

- Bioinformatics

Background

Better alternatives for repair of the bladder, urethra, and pelvic floor will involve tissue-engineering techniques that attempt to recapitulate normal organ function. Diseased bladder, urethral, and pelvic floor tissues have traditionally been replaced or repaired with tissues harvested from other sites of the body or transplanted from another body. However, these approaches rarely replace the entire function of the original tissue. For example, current bladder reconstructive procedures use tissue from the patient's own gastrointestinal tract. This is a complicated surgical procedure associated with significant complications, including infection, intestinal obstruction, mucus production, electrolyte abnormalities, perforation, and cancer. When reconstructed reservoirs become dysfunctional, a surgical procedure called bladder augmentation is required. These potential side effects have impelled researchers to develop new technologies in the field of tissue engineering.

In other disease states, such as urinary incontinence or vesicoureteral reflux, artificial agents (e.g., Teflon paste and silicone micro-particles) have been used as bulking substances; however, these substances are not entirely biocompatible.

Engineered tissues are critically needed to replace or repair lost and functionally deficient genitourinary organs. Cells may or may not be needed for tissue regeneration. If cells are needed, then several sources may be available, including

- Autologous cells—cells that occur naturally in a person's body

- Heterologous cells—cells derived from another source

- Mature stem cells

- Progenitor stem cells

Stem cell populations associated with the urinary tract have been recently identified, although their characterization is incomplete. Stem cells have been classically defined as a subpopulation of cells that are present in self-renewing tissues and responsible for the long-term maintenance and acute repair of the organ. The main criteria used to identify such cells are as follows:

- Slow-cycling

- High *in vivo* and *in vitro* proliferative potential

- Cytological and ultra-structural features

- Expression of certain "stem cell markers"

- Well-protected location and specialized "stem cell niche"

- Associations with predominant sites of tumor initiation

Recent findings have shown that stem cells are also present in some tissues that have not been traditionally regarded as self-renewing, such as tissues of the liver, brain, and heart. Moreover, unexpected flexibility in some stem cell populations has been demonstrated, including the ability of hematopoietic and mesenchymal stem cells to be directed to the formation of other cell types, such as smooth muscle cells. Stem cells can also be derived from embryos and from nuclear transfer using somatic cells.

Stem cells are classified according to the types of cells they are capable of producing. Unipotent stem cells produce a single fixed type of daughter cell; multipotent stem cells produce several fixed types of daughter cells; and pluripotent stem cells do not have a fixed potential for development. Pluripotent stem cells are capable of generating different cell types of single or multiple organs or tissues.

The completion of several large-scale sequencing projects has provided the genomic sequences for humans and several other species. This is an extraordinary opportunity to discover and characterize genes and gene groups that play important roles in regulatory pathways and biological processes such as the development of the bladder and its response to injury and disease. Elucidating the genetic program changes that are associated with normal maturation or pathologic alterations within the bladder will lead to hypotheses that can be tested using genetic, biochemical, and pharmacological analyses. This, in turn, will catalyze and form the basis of future advances at all levels of bladder, urethral, and pelvic floor research.

Cost and Impact

The financial costs associated with loss of tissue function in the bladder, urethra, and pelvic floor are estimated to amount to tens of billions of dollars. The societal costs are enormous. People with congenital and acquired bladder and urethral disease frequently have chronic

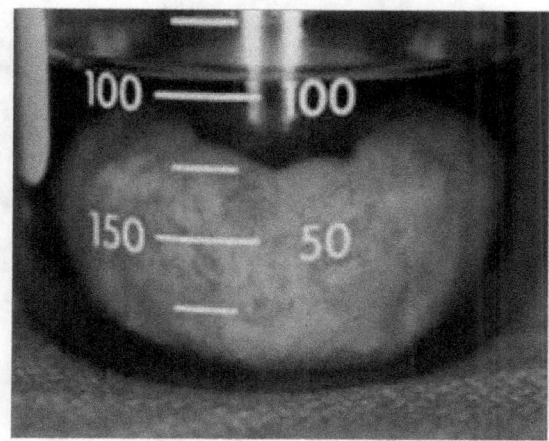

A bladder engineered in the laboratory. *(Photo Credit: Dr. Anthony Atala, Children's Hopital and Harvard Medical School.)*

abnormalities that require long-term health care and that could lead to disease in other organ systems. Diagnostic techniques and tissue engineering techniques for treatments that use either autologous cells or stem cells could provide better long-term solutions for people suffering from bladder and urethral disease.

Congenital and acquired defects of the lower urinary tract result in the bladder's inability to function as a low-pressure storage and emptying vehicle. This results in reduced bladder elasticity and urinary incontinence with subsequent deterioration of the upper urinary tract. More than 50,000 people are diagnosed with bladder cancer each year according to the American Cancer Society, and a subset of them requires surgical removal of the bladder (cystectomy). More than 15,000 people per year may benefit from research that develops improved techniques for bladder replacement.

New tissue engineering, stem cell, and genomic technologies could have a great impact on the health care of more than 13 million Americans who have urinary incontinence and the subset of that population that has disorders of the urethra and pelvic floor, problems that lead to increased morbidity and poor quality of life.

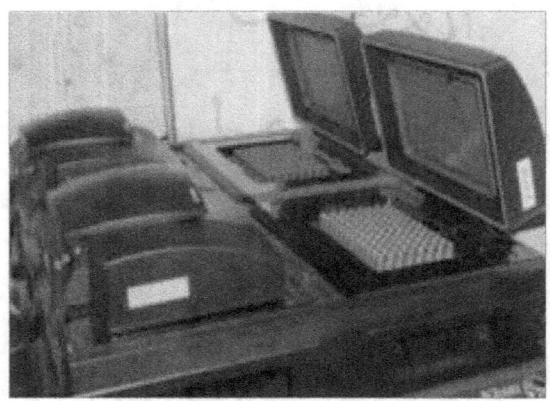

A Tetrad PCR Machine used for setting up polymerase chain reactions (PCR). The machine makes multiple copies of DNA from scarce genes. (Photo Credit: Harvard Medical School/Partners Healthcare System for Genetics and Genomics and Biopolymers Facility Sequencing Core.)

The application of gene expression profiling technologies to normal and genetically or experimentally modified bladders would allow

- Insight into coordinate regulation and would coordinate function among groups of molecules

- Characterization of novel genes and proteins involved in carrying out specific biologic processes

- Improved understanding of regulatory cascades and the biologic processes themselves

- Ability to profile the effects of an individual gene, a drug, an injury, or a hormone on the bladder

The development of new technologies for biomedicine would have a great impact on how studies of the bladder, urethra, and pelvic floor are conducted. Current technologies have the primary limitation of low throughput, which means that the number of tests that can be performed in a given period of time is low. This especially hampers the study of biologically heterogeneous disorders in humans. Additionally, current research tools for analyzing nucleic acids and proteins rely on large sample sizes. This limits the application of these tools in both humans and small animal models where starting material is limited.

What the polymerase chain reaction (PCR) has done for research over the last 10 years will be equaled by the development of new high throughput technologies that allow the analysis of large numbers of specimens with minimal volume and the ability to analyze increasingly smaller populations of pure cells. These technologies could lead to great advancements in the understanding of congenital and acquired disorders of the bladder and play a role in the development of new drugs and therapies.

The engineering of bladder, urethral, and pelvic floor tissues and structures, either for complete replacement or for augmentation of organ function, would be advantageous for a large number of disease states. The engineering of tissues could be performed with biomaterials or cells alone for smaller defects or with biomaterials with cells for larger deficiencies. The cells could be autologous, heterologous, or from stem cell sources. Bioengineering technologies could provide an available repository of tissues for revitalization of the lower urinary tract.

Identification of urologic stem cells is of major importance because

- Urologic stem cells may be the targets of chemical and viral oncogenesis (development and growth of neoplasms—abnormal tissue that proliferates rapidly) and could therefore be a predominant source of malignancy that may lead to neoplastic conditions such as bladder and prostate cancer

- A deficiency of urologic stem cells may lead to a variety of tissue abnormalities, including acquired abnormalities such as hypercontractile bladders and developmental abnormalities involving the ureteric bud, urogenital sinus, and müllerian and wolffian structures

- Urologic stem cells may be ideal targets for gene therapy

- Urologic stem cells may play a major role in wound repair secondary to injury or in acquired inflammatory conditions such as interstitial cystitis

- Urologic stem cells may be needed for the construction of artificial tissues and organs

Development and applications of tissue bioengineering techniques using stem cells could enable people to "self-donate" an organ such as a bladder. Non-diseased cells could be harvested from the patient and grown into a full or partial organ in the laboratory, which would then be transplanted into the donor. All people with bladder disease could benefit from advances in the areas of genomics, tissue engineering, and stem cells.

Current Research and Opportunities

Current extramural and intramural research on bladder genomics, tissue engineering, and stem cells funded by the National Institutes of Health (NIH) includes studies on the bioengineering of bladder tissue, novel scaffolds for bladder replacement, muscle-cell-mediated gene therapy for incontinence, gene-environment interactions (Odyssey cohort), comparison of *in vivo* and *in vitro*

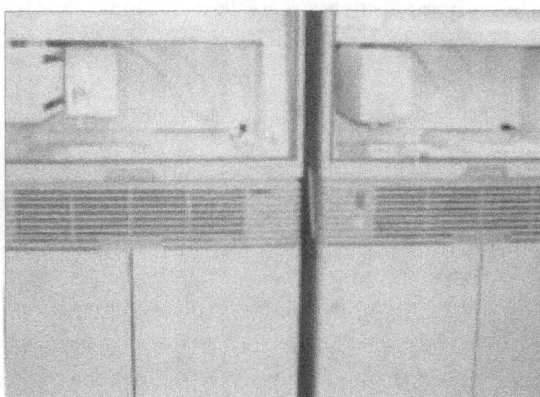

ABI 3700 Capillary Electrophoresis Units Sequencing Instruments used to determine the sequence of amino acids in DNA. (Photo Credit: Harvard Medical School/Partners Healthcare System for Genetics and Genomics and Biopolymers Facility Sequencing Core.)

tissue engineering, and genetic susceptibility to bladder cancer. Research opportunities exist in genomics, stem cells, cell signaling and regulation, tissue engineering, biomechanics, bioinformatics, gene therapy, and genetic engineering.

Genomics

The completion of several large-scale sequencing projects has provided the genomic sequences for a number of species, including humans. This affords an extraordinary opportunity to discover and characterize genes and gene groups that play important roles in regulatory pathways and biological processes such as the development of the bladder and its response to injury and disease. Applying expression-profiling strategies to the various cellular compartments (e.g., epithelium, smooth muscle, and stromal tissue) within the bladder and urethra could be especially informative. Technologies to accomplish this are emerging and include laser capture microdissection (LCM) and fluorescence-activated cell sorting (FACS).

However, because of the current amounts of RNA needed for expression profiling using microarrays, these approaches, especially LCM, may be limited to the use of PCR-based approaches designed to examine selected gene products or to look for mutations or polymorphisms in candidate genes. In addition, FACS requires the availability of specific cell surface markers or fluorescently labeled cells. Attention should be given to genes with known significance in development, proliferation, and differentiation and maintenance of smooth muscle cells or of bladder epithelium. This includes growth factors, cell-signaling components, oncogenes (genes that normally encode proteins involved in cell growth or regulation), and transcription factors (factors involved in transferring genetic code information from one kind of nucleic acid to another).

Genomics and proteomics may also help characterize the sequence of events that occur during bladder regeneration. For example, genomic analysis of tissue samples

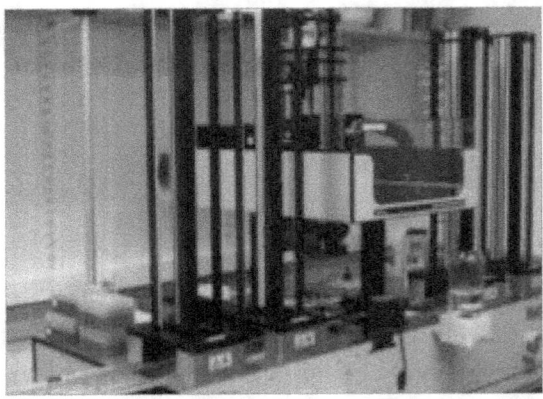

A Packard Monotrack Robot, designed for high throughoutput screening of randomly selected compounds for a defined assay, for example, testing the function of specific proteins, drugs, and antibodies. (Photo Credit: Harvard Medical School/Partners Healthcare System for Genetics and Genomics and Biopolymers Facility Sequencing Core.)

from regenerated tissue at different points in time could characterize global gene expression. Similar studies of proteins found in the tissue as well as in the urine could be used for proteomics. Additionally, the gene-expression profile and proteomic "fingerprint" of each cell type that regenerates could be obtained. These fingerprints could then be compared to "normal" cells as well as to the "abnormal" cells from which they were obtained.

Genomics and proteomics will play a large role in defining what happens to all types of bladder cells once they are placed in culture. Future research should

- Identify changes in gene expression profiles in a normal setting versus a pathological setting and in developmentally recapitulated tissue using tissue-engineering techniques. Knowledge gained may lead to future studies of transgenic- or virus-based approaches that target relevant growth or differentiation modulators to selected bladder compartments.

- Design a therapeutic strategy to alter interactions between epithelial cells and connective tissue cells within the bladder microenvironment. For example, reducing or preventing tumor progression by altering the expression of a gene involved in epithelial cell proliferation may be possible.

- Identify the underlying genetic program(s) involved in the initiation and progression of many pathological conditions, particularly if animal models can be developed.

- Study the progression of bladder disease from normal to end-stage disease—a critical study that requires establishing reproducible and acceptable animal models.

- Conduct clinical studies to acquire epidemiological data regarding familial patterns of occurrence of bladder, urethral, and pelvic floor disease. These families could then be analyzed to seek out the genetic bases of these disorders.

- Identify persons with a predisposition for disease to assure early intervention.

- Develop genomic and proteomic databases that specifically address cells of the lower urinary tract, including epithelium; bladder smooth muscle; fibroblasts (cells capable of producing collagen) in the lamina propria (the layer of connective tissue underlying the epithelium of a mucous membrane), the pelvic floor, and the perimysium. (the fibrous sheath surrounding smooth muscles); myofibroblasts (cells that have some properties of smooth muscle such as contractility and are thought to be involved in the contracture of wounds); and urethral sphincter cells. Once these data sets are developed, cell-type-specific chip arrays can be prepared and used to profile these subsets of genes in normal and diseased bladders.

- Apply state-of-the-art genomic approaches such as laser capture microscopy, tissue arrays, and mass spectroscopy to the study of the complex mixed tissue types of the lower urinary tract. Information obtained using these tools will enhance the ability to design therapies. For example, drug treatments could be designed based on the receptor content and signaling pathways discovered in this way.

Stem Cells, Cell Regulation, and Cell Signaling

During the past 20 years, remarkable progress has been made in elucidating the tissue interactions and molecules that regulate the formation of the bladder, urethra, and pelvic floor. From this work, it is now clear that interactions between the epithelium and mesenchyme are essential for the formation of normal tissues and organs. These seminal discoveries may soon be exploited to generate sizable quantities of tissue suitable for study and transplantation, provided that strategies can be developed to isolate, expand, and differentiate native autologous cells and stem cells *in vitro* and *in vivo*.

Cell signaling occurs during normal and abnormal bladder development. The cellular signaling or growth factors required to regenerate normal functional bladder tissue are not known. Research on cell signaling in the bladder should

- Focus on understanding the mechanism of bladder regeneration.

- Elucidate further the cell signaling that occurs between the epithelium and smooth muscle of the bladder and the role of extrinsic growth factors and their receptors. This knowledge will direct future biomaterial development.

- Define further the immunobiology of biomaterials used for tissue engineering.

- Define the effects of biomaterials on the surrounding normal tissue.

- Determine the role of hormones, growth factors, and cytokines (hormone-like proteins that regulate the duration and intensity of the immune response and mediate cell-to-cell communication) present in the biomaterials used for tissue regeneration.

- Determine how the mechanism of tissue regeneration differs from normal wound healing.

Understanding the cell signaling mechanisms occurring during tissue regeneration is crucial if engineering technology is to develop a viable alternative for bladder, urethra, and pelvic floor repair. Furthermore, the stem cell biology of the bladder, urethra, and pelvic floor is largely unknown. Research should

- Define the features and location of these stem cells.

- Establish reproducible conditions and protocols for identifying, retrieving, and maintaining stem cells.

- Use several approaches to identify and isolate bladder, urethral, and pelvic floor stem cells, including the use of cell-specific markers to sort putative stem cells from tissues; the evaluation of *in vitro* and *in vivo* growth and differentiation capabilities; and the use of morphologic, molecular, and clonigenic (the ability of a stem cell population to be derived from a single cell) assays.

- Establish the lineage relationship between disparate cell types.

- Identify signaling molecules that direct decisions concerning stem cell fate.

- Generate monoclonal antibodies and complementary DNA (cDNA) probes that discriminate between pluripotent stem cells and developmental intermediary epithelial, vascular, and mesenchymal progenitor cell types.

- Develop novel approaches to characterization, such as using microarray methods to determine the profile of expressed genes.

- Define the developmental potential of bladder, urethral, and pelvic floor stem cells, and the properties of immediate committed daughter cells. For example, which stem cells are present in adult tissues? When and how do stem cells generate epithelial, mesenchymal, and vascular progenitors? What is the normal function of these stem cells in urologic organs? What is the role of these stem cells in maintaining homeostasis in self-renewing cell populations?

- Employ current fate-mapping techniques (i.e., retro-viral-mediated gene transfer approaches) to address the above questions.

- Determine functional genomics, including gene expression profiling and surface markers.

A variety of adult organs have been identified as containing stem cells that may be sufficiently pluripotent to generate cells in organs other than the ones from which they were derived. For instance, bone marrow stem cells could be induced to differentiate into smooth muscle cells. These findings need to be documented further and to be applied rigorously to the identification of bladder, urethral, and pelvic floor stem cells. Research needs to

- Define the genes controlling stem cell division (asymmetric and symmetric) and the commitment of progeny to a particular fate.

- Determine the interaction of these cells with the microenvironment that helps define its stem origin.

Once stem cells have been identified, they can be injected into normal and dysfunctional tissue. These cells could be genetically modified to provide or enhance expression of a depleted growth factor. Furthermore, these cells could accelerate recovery processes and enhance repair of the bladder, urethra, or pelvic floor.

The role of tissue engineering and stem cells in bladder, urethral, and pelvic floor disease needs to be defined. The engineered tissues or stem cells could be therapeutic targets for gene therapy, and their activity could be modulated for therapeutic benefit, in combination with radiotherapy and chemotherapy, for a variety of bladder conditions, including neoplasia (rapid, abnormal cell growth) and inflammatory disease.

Tissue Engineering

Advances in cell biology and cell research will enable scientists to grow tissues and organs in the laboratory starting from only a few cells. For example, under the appropriate conditions, cells could theoretically be "instructed" to develop into a bladder. This would eliminate many of the current obstacles to organ replacement, such as donor-recipient mismatches and limited organ availability. Future research studies should attempt to

- Define the conditions required for the formation of bladder, urethral, and pelvic floor tissues and organs. Tissue formation has been established as being dependent on the presence of organ-specific cells and biocompatible matrices; however, the full extent of tissue-inducing parameters remains to be identified.

- Determine the precise role of the cells in the formation of tissues and organs.

- Determine the possible role of blood vessel and nerve elements in regulating tissue and organ formation.

- Develop minimal functional parameters necessary to produce functional tissue replacements.

- Develop models of long-term remodeling and engineered tissue survival to minimize costly animal trials.

- Develop an *in vitro* (test tube) model to minimize the costly *in vivo* (animal) testing and development that is involved in the complex remodeling process.

- Develop instrumentation for minimally invasive diagnosis of lower urinary tract disorders involving biomechanical assessment, functional imaging, and urodynamics.

Novel technologies capable of capturing the developmental potential of the cells need to be explored. Future research should

- Develop methods to manipulate the local environment (through the scaffold material, extracellular matrix, or appropriate growth factors) to induce the controlled regeneration of tissues or organs starting from these cells.

- Explore further the effect of the bladder biomechanical properties on early regeneration.

- Determine cell production capabilities and cellular function tools.

- Define and standardize biomaterials and their desirable material properties (e.g., elasticity and intrinsic growth factors) with the appropriate degradation profile.

- Explore the use of material chemistry or its micro and macro structure to increase re-vascularization and to promote normal regeneration. The addition of bioactive groups or other functional groups to allow improved interactions with peptides or proteins to enable tuning of the tissue scaffolds may be needed to achieve a specific cellular response.

- Establish biomaterial preparation and scaffold production and standardization laboratories.

- Explore novel technologies capable of capturing the developmental potential of the cells.

- Define methods of manipulating the local environment (through the scaffold material, extracellular matrix, or appropriate growth factors) to induce the controlled regeneration of tissues or organs starting from these cells.

- Develop cell production capabilities and cellular function tools.

- Integrate desirable material properties (e.g., elasticity) with the appropriate degradation profile.

Bioinformatics

The subject of emerging technologies brings special issues to the bladder, urethra, and pelvic floor. The past 10 years have seen dramatic advances in the development of instrumentation for the study of molecular biology. Completion of the human genome brings about new challenges for applying this wealth of data. As a part of this effort, there has been a resurgence of interest in the application of technologies for the study of proteins. LCM and the development of cDNA microarray analysis of gene expression offer the ability to define the gene expression patterns of individual tissue types. These technologies all focus on using smaller samples of material for discovery research. The development of newer techniques that may define individual small cell populations would be a significant advance in the dissection of bladder, urethra, and pelvic floor tissues into functional elements.

Current challenges include (1) determining the progression to disease and (2) collecting tissue specimens that would define this spectrum. To accomplish this, adequate animal model systems of the bladder, urethra, and pelvic floor need to be developed. The bladder and urethra consist of an innervated, complex, muscular layer lined with epithelium. Most model systems poorly replicate this system, failing to correctly mimic the extrinsic processes present within these organ systems. Cell populations that need to be addressed include epithelium, fibroblasts, myoblasts (primitive muscle cells with the potential for developing into a muscle fiber), and contractile cells of the bladder, urethra, and pelvic floor, as well as the non-cellular components of these organs.

Future research projects should endeavor to

- Define the changes that occur in the progression to disease rather than in end-stage disease states.

- Develop resources around cell types in the bladder, urethra, and pelvic floor, including cDNA and protein profiles of these cell types.

- Make available and refine technologies that will isolate and study as individual components the functionally separate cell populations of the bladder, urethra, and pelvic floor.

- Define the mechanisms by which extrinsic processes affect the cell populations of these organ systems.

- Define the factors that predispose people to disease.

Bioinformatics is expected to play a major role in bladder and urethral genomics, tissue engineering, stem cell research, and clinical application. Self-renewing stem cells usually originate from a rare multipotent cell population. During the engineering of tissue structures, genome-wide gene expression analyses should be performed to define regulatory pathways in bladder cells and their global genetic programs. Subtracted cDNA libraries from native bladder and stem cell populations should be analyzed with bioinformatic and array hybridization strategies.

A large percentage of the several thousand gene products that would be characterized are expected to correspond to previously undescribed molecules, some involved in regulatory functions. As the research in the area of tissue engineering and stem cells proceeds, the ability to rapidly access previously observed cell behavior would prove valuable. This behavior will be a function of the cell's environmental context, and it should be tracked at the levels of molecular expression and whole-cell responses. In this way, data can be aggregated to predict cell responses and, thereby, to control cell roles in tissue regeneration.

These sets of complete data should be made available in biologic process-oriented databases, representing the molecular phenotype of specific cell populations. Training and equipment in the area of bioinformatics will be needed to accomplish the above. In addition, access to deposited searchable databases generated from bladder-associated microarray and proteomic studies must be made available to the scientific community. These efforts should be coordinated with current NIH committees working on functional genomic and bioinformatics initiatives.

A considerable infrastructure is required to support the genomic approaches listed above. This includes a bioinformatics unit to assist with database mining, gene discovery, sequence analysis, and expression analysis. Access to computer systems, database infrastructure, and direct-user support for the identification and characterization of genes under study is important as well. Advanced commercial high-throughput technologies are available and include commercial microarray systems and subtraction cDNA methods.

Gene Therapy and Genetic Engineering

Technologies such as gene therapy and genetic engineering are also essential for the eventual use of tissue engineering and stem cell technologies in treating the spectrum of diseases affecting the bladder, urethra, and pelvic floor. An appropriate focus is expected in these areas of research.

Research Requirements

Workforce

The development of emerging technologies is currently hampered by the lack of appropriately trained investigators. Currently, new technologies that would most likely yield the greatest impact are not taught well, and few training programs provide students with in-depth skills to perform this research. In addition, few students are interested in acquiring these skills. Cooperation and coordination with other NIH initiatives must be fostered.

Several training awards should be directed to the fields of bladder and urethral genomics, tissue engineering, and stem cell research. These awards may be given to

- Train newly independent scientists who can demonstrate the need for a period of intensive research focus as a means of enhancing their research directives in the areas of bladder, urethral, and pelvic floor genomics, tissue engineering, or stem cell research

- Train research scientists who have identified a mentor with extensive experience in bladder, urethral, and pelvic floor genomics, tissue engineering, or stem cell research

- Train health scientists who have the opportunity to receive research training in the areas of bladder, urethral, and pelvic floor genomics, tissue engineering, or stem cell research

- Train or provide supplemental funding to outstanding scientists who have demonstrated a sustained level of productivity and whose expertise, research accomplishments, and contributions to the field have been, and will continue to be, critical to the mission outlined in this report

Infrastructure

Successful applications of bladder, urethral, and pelvic floor genomics, tissue engineering, or stem cell research should be pursued through NIH-solicited and investigator-initiated research programs, training, and scientist awards. Multi-centered and program research centers should be established. The use of genomic-based technologies is of major importance. Furthermore, understanding the basic processes that control stem cell progeny will facilitate new approaches to wound repair and the creation of tissues and organs for transplantation.

In addition, clinical applications for tissue engineering and stem cells will improve preventive and therapeutic approaches, including gene transfer, for a wide range of bladder, urethral, and pelvic floor diseases. Examples include cancer, functional disorders, end-stage organ disease, and congenital abnormalities. Thus, findings generated from this research will be highly relevant to many NIH components.

Tissue and Specimen Banks

The development of appropriate tissue and specimen banks containing paraffin-embedded and frozen tissues is essential for the application of these technologies. Because they are aimed at high-throughput, statistically relevant conclusions, many technological approaches are dependent on samples from large populations. Some technologies will be able to use both the cellular components and the free proteins for analysis, a freely available benefit that will require the development of registries and core storage facilities to identify appropriate people for study.

With highest priority, a bladder, urethral, and pelvic floor primary and stem cell bank should be established that would include a depository and central distribution center for sharing cells, reagents, and model systems. An academic center with access to human and animal urologic tissue sources would be preferable as a selected site. The primary and stem cell and reagent bank would operate under the auspices of the National Institute of Diabetes and Digestive and Kidney Diseases (NIDDK) of the NIH.

Interactions with Pharmaceutical/Biotechnology Companies

Interactions with the biotechnology and large pharmaceutical industries should be encouraged. These industries have the research and development budgets to support the extensive equipment and specialized personnel cost incumbent with this research. They also have dedicated resources that they seek to use. Additionally, pharmaceutical and biotechnology companies are well motivated to study these processes because they are primarily chronic and affect an aging population. Technology development is expected to drive biological discovery for the next decade.

Public Interest and Educational Efforts

As the sciences of bladder, urethral, and pelvic floor genomics, tissue engineering, and stem cells continue to be developed, scientists should not overlook particular experimental therapies that could raise ethical concerns among some members of the public. Although the scientific rationale for a particular type of research may be quite clear to researchers, it could be quite controversial to the public as a whole. Forums that discuss the ethical, legal, and social issues in biomedical research should guide policy decisions in these areas. These forums include

- The NIH Office of Biotechnology Activities
- The NIH Office for Protection from Research Risks
- The President's National Bioethics Advisory Committee

Ongoing communication among scientists, physicians, educators, ethicists, theologians, elected officials, and the public is essential to guide the future of this research and to ensure that America continues to invest judiciously and responsibly in biomedical research.

Ongoing Review and Advisory Groups

The NIDDK should hold workshops to discuss scientific issues relevant to bladder, urethral, and pelvic floor genomics, tissue engineering, and stem cell research. These workshops should also include discussions regarding inter-institutional collaborations that would further advance research in these areas.

A mechanism should be established within the NIDDK to coordinate all endeavors in bladder, urethral, and pelvic floor genomics, tissue engineering, and stem cell research and to ensure proper development, oversight, and evaluation of established guidelines.

PHARMACOLOGY

Recommendations

The Bladder Research Progress Review Group made the following recommendations for future research in pharmacology of the lower urinary tract, in order of priority:

- ⤵ Develop drugs that can modulate bladder sensory pathways in the peripheral and central nervous systems, including drugs that mediate visceral pain.

- ⤵ Develop specific drugs that can modulate the micturition (voiding) threshold in the central nervous system.

- ⤵ Develop orally administered smooth-muscle-specific agents for treatment of lower urinary tract smooth-muscle disease, including overactive bladder (myogenic origin) and contractile failure.

- ⤵ Develop drugs that protect peripheral post-ganglionic nerves from degeneration (neuroprotective drugs) and drugs that can stimulate nerve growth and regeneration. (These drugs would be useful in the treatment of diseases such as diabetes, bladder obstruction, and degenerative diseases of the nervous system such as multiple sclerosis)

- ⤵ Develop drugs that can affect the properties of urinary tract epithelium, including drugs that can alter the arachidonic acid cascade involved in the inflammatory process, causing symptoms of urinary urgency, frequency, and pain.

- ⤵ Develop drugs to improve blood flow to the bladder, possibly by stimulating angiogenesis (development of blood vessels).

- ⤵ Develop novel chronic drug delivery systems, including administration of drugs directly into the bladder (intravesical administration).

- ⤵ Develop drugs to regulate connective tissue matrix synthesis and degradation.

Benjamin Franklin to John Franklin The Flexible Catheter

Philadelphia, December 8, 1752

Dear Brother,

Reflecting yesterday on your Desire to have a flexible Catheter, a Thought struck into my Mind how one might possibly be made: And lest you should not readily conceive it by any Description of mine, I went immediately to the Silversmith's, and gave Directions for making one, (sitting by 'till it was finish'd), that it might be ready for this Post. But now it is done I have some Apprehensions that it may be too large to be easy: if so, a Silversmith can easily make it less, by twisting it on a smaller Wire, and putting a smaller Pipe to the End, if the Pipe be really necessary. This Machine may either be cover'd with a small fine Gut first clean'd and soak'd a Night in a Solution of Alum and Salt in Water, then rubb'd dry which will preserve it longer from Putrefaction; then wet again, and drawn on, and ty'd to the Pipes at each End where little Hollows are made for the Thread to bind in and the Surface greas'd; Or perhaps it may be used without the Gut, having only a little Tallow rubb'd over it, to smooth it and fill the Joints. I think it is as flexible as could be expected in a thing of the kind, and I imagine will readily comply with the Turns of the Passage, yet has Stiffness enough to be protruded; if not, the enclos'd Wire may be us'd to stiffen the hinder Part of the Pipe while the fore Part is push'd forward; and as it proceeds the Wire may be gradually withdrawn. The Tube is of such a Nature, that when you have Occasion to withdraw it its Diameter will lessen, whereby it will move more easily. It is also a kind of Scrue, and may be both withdrawn and introduc'd by turning. Experience is necessary for the right using of all new Tools or Instruments, and that will perhaps suggest some Improvements to this Instrument as well as better direct the Manner of Using it.

I have read Whytt on Lime Water. You desire my Thoughts on what he says. But what can I say? He relates Facts and Experiments; and they must be allow'd good, if not contradicted by other Facts and Experiments. May not one guess by holding Lime Water some time in one's Mouth, whether it is likely to injure the Bladder?

I know not what to advise, either as to the Injection, or the Operation. I can only pray God to direct you for the best, and to grant Success.

I am, my dear Brother Yours most affectionately

I find Whytt's Experiments are approv'd and recommended by Dr. Mead.

From The Writings of Benjamin Franklin, Volume II: Philadelphia, 1726 - 1757

EXECUTIVE COMMITTEE

CHAIR: **Linda Dairiki Shortliffe, M.D.**
Chair, Department of Urology
Stanford University School of Medicine
Stanford, California

William C. de Groat, Ph.D.
Department of Pharmacology
University of Pittsburgh School of Medicine
Pittsburgh, Pennsylvania

John O. DeLancey, M.D.
Department of Obstetrics and Gynecology
University of Michigan
Ann Arbor, Michigan

Monica Liebert, Ph.D.
Director of Research
American Urological Association, Inc.
Baltimore, Maryland

John D. McConnell, M.D.
Chairman, Department of Urology
University of Texas Southwestern Medical Center
Dallas, Texas

Vicki Ratner, M.D.
NIDDK Advisory Council Member
President, Interstitial Cystitis Association
Rockville, Maryland

Anthony J. Schaeffer, M.D.
Chairman, Department of Urology
Northwestern University Medical School
Chicago, Illinois

William D. Steers, M.D.
Chair, Department of Urology
University of Virginia
Health Sciences Center
Charlottesville, Virginia

Dana Weaver-Osterholtz, M.D.
Clinical Associate Professor
University of Missouri
Columbia, Missouri

WORK AND FOCUS GROUPS

Group 1:

Diabetes, Cancer, Development

Diabetes

Chairs: Michael Chancellor, Robert Weiss

Jeanette Brown

George Christ

William de Groat

Susan Keay

Edward Macarak

Anthony Schaeffer

Michael Siroky

Ann Stapleton

Jeremy Tuttle

Dana Weaver-Osterholtz

Ursula Wesselman

Cancer

Chair: Edward Messing

Harris Foster

Stephen Hewitt

Edmund Lattime

Monica Liebert

Vicki Ratner

Ricardo Saban

Michael Sacks

Tung-Tien Sun

Development

Chairs: Larry Baskin, Ananias Diokno

James Ashton-Miller

Anthony Atala

Linda Brubaker

Toby Chai

John DeLancey

Philip Hanno

Anna Herzog

Barry Kogan

Bradley Kropp

James Lessard

Robert Levin

Peggy Norton

Neil Resnick

Brenda Russell

Linda Shortliffe

William Steers

Group 2:

Incontinence

Chairs: Linda Brubaker, Peggy Norton

James Ashton-Miller

Larry Baskin

Toby Chai

George Christ

John DeLancey

Anna Herzog

Neil Resnick

William Steers

Jeremy Tuttle

Emerging Technologies

Chairs: Anthony Atala, Bradley Kropp

Michael Chancellor

Stephen Hewitt

James Lessard

Monica Liebert

Edward Macarak

Brenda Russell

Michael Sacks

Tung-Tien Sun

Inflammation/Infection/Interstitial Cystitis

Chairs: Philip Hanno, Anthony Schaeffer,
Ann Stapleton

Jeanette Brown

Ananias Diokno

Harris Foster

Susan Keay

Edmund Lattime

Edward Messing

Vicki Ratner

Ricardo Saban

Michael Siroky

Ursula Wesselman

Obstruction

Chair: Barry Kogan

William de Groat

Robert Levin

Linda Shortliffe

William Steers

Dana Weaver-Osterholtz

Robert Weiss

Group 3:

Epithelium, Muscle, Nerve/Vascular,
Connective tissue/Matrix

Epithelium

Chairs: Susan Keay, Tung-Tien Sun

Anthony Atala

Philip Hanno

Stephen Hewitt

Edmund Lattime

Edward Messing

Vicki Ratner

Anthony Schaeffer

Ann Stapleton

Robert Weiss

Muscle

Chairs: George Christ, Harris Foster

James Ashton-Miller

John DeLancey

Ananias Diokno

Anna Herzog

Barry Kogan

James Lessard

Neil Resnick

Brenda Russell

Linda Shortliffe

Nerve/Vascular

Chairs: Toby Chai, Jeremy Tuttle

Michael Chancellor

William de Groat

Robert Levin

Ricardo Saban

Michael Siroky

William Steers

Ursula Wesselman

Connective Tissue/Matrix

Chair: Edward Macarak

Larry Baskin

Linda Brubaker

Jeanette Brown

Bradley Kropp

Monica Liebert

Peggy Norton

Michael Sacks

Dana Weaver-Osterholtz

Focus Groups:

Clinical Trials, Epidemiology, Pharmacology

Clinical Trials

Chairs: Linda Shortliffe, William Steers

James Ashton-Miller

Anthony Atala

Larry Baskin

Ananias Diokno

Harris Foster

Barry Kogan

Bradley Kropp

Edmund Lattime

Edward Messing

Peggy Norton

Vicki Ratner

Michael Sacks

Anthony Schaeffer

Linda Shortliffe

Michael Siroky

William Steers

Dana Weaver-Osterholtz

Robert Weiss

Epidemiology

Chairs: Jeanette Brown, Anna Herzog

John DeLancey

Philip Hanno

Susan Keay

Monica Liebert

Neil Resnick

Ann Stapleton

Pharmacology

Chair: Robert Levin

Linda Brubaker

Toby Chai

Michael Chancellor

George Christ

William de Groat

Stephen Hewitt

James Lessard

Edward Macarak

Brenda Russell

Ricardo Saban

Tung-Tien Sun

Jeremy Tuttle

Ursula Wesselman

PARTICIPANTS

James Ashton-Miller, Ph.D.
Distinguished Research Scientist
Biomechanics Research Laboratory
University of Michigan
Ann Arbor, MI

Anthony Atala, M.D.
Associate Professor of Surgery
Division of Urology
Harvard/Children's Hospital
Boston, MA

Larry Baskin, M.D.
Chief, Pediatric Urology
University of California-San Francisco
San Francisco, CA

Lisa Begg, Dr.PH
Director of Research Programs
Office of Research on Women's Health
National Institutes of Health
Bethesda, MD

Frank Bellino, Ph.D.
Program Administrator
Endocrinology Branch
National Institute on Aging
National Institutes of Health
Bethesda, MD

Carolyn Vogel Benson
Writer-Editor
Division of Kidney, Urologic,
and Hematologic Diseases
National Institute of Diabetes and
Digestive and Kidney Diseases
National Institutes of Health
Bethesda, MD

Josephine P. Briggs, M.D.
Director
Division of Kidney, Urologic,
and Hematologic Diseases
National Institute of Diabetes and
Digestive and Kidney Diseases
National Institutes of Health
Bethesda, MD

Jeanette S. Brown, M.D.
Professor
Department of Obstetrics, Gynecology,
and Reproductive Sciences
Epidemiology and Biostatistics
Director, Women's Continence Center
University of California, San Francisco
San Francisco, CA

Linda Brubaker, M.D.
Professor and Fellowship Director
Department of Obstetrics and Gynecology
Loyola University Medical Center
Maywood, IL

Toby Chai, M.D.
Assistant Professor
Division of Urology
University of Maryland
Baltimore, MD

Jodi Chappell
American Urogynecologic Society
Manager, Congressional and Regulatory Affairs
Smith, Bucklin, and Associates,
Health Care Practice Group
Washington, DC

Michael B. Chancellor, M.D.
Professor
University of Pittsburgh
Pittsburgh, PA

George Christ, Ph.D.
Professor
Albert Einstein College of Medicine
Bronx, NY

William C. de Groat, Ph.D.
Professor of Pharmacology
Department of Pharmacology
University of Pittsburgh School of Medicine
Pittsburgh, PA

John O. DeLancey, M.D.
Norman F. Miller Professor
Department of Obstetrics and Gynecology
University of Michigan Medical Center
Ann Arbor, MI

Ananias Diokno, M.D.
Chief, Department of Urology
William Beaumont Hospital
Royal Oak, MI

Richard Farishian, Ph.D.
Deputy Director
Office of Scientific Program and Policy Analysis
National Institute of Diabetes and
Digestive and Kidney Diseases
National Institutes of Health
Bethesda, MD

Harris E. Foster, M.D.
Associate Professor of Surgery
Section of Urology
Yale University School of Medicine
New Haven, CT

Cheryl Gartley
President and Founder
The Simon Foundation for Continence
Wilmette, DE

Philip M. Hanno, M.D.
Division of Urology
University of Pennsylvania
Philadelphia, PA

Mary M. Harris
Writer-Editor
Office of Communications and Public Liaison
National Institute of Diabetes and
Digestive and Kidney Diseases
National Institutes of Health
Bethesda, MD

Anna R. Herzog, Ph.D.
Senior Research Scientist
Institute for Social Research
University of Michigan
Ann Arbor, MI

Stephen Hewitt, M.D., Ph.D.
Clinical Investigator
Laboratory of Pathology
National Cancer Institute
National Institutes of Health
Bethesda, MD

Stephen P. Heyse, M.D., M.P.H.
Medical Officer
National Institute of Allergy and Infectious Diseases
National Institutes of Health
Bethesda, MD

Susan Keay, M.D., Ph.D.
Associate Professor of Medicine
Department of Medicine
Division of Infectious Diseases
University of Maryland School of Medicine
Baltimore, MD

Barry Kogan, M.D.
Chief, Division of Urology
Albany Medical College
Albany, NY

Bradley Kropp, M.D.
Associate Professor of Urology
Department of Urology
University of Oklahoma Health Sciences Center
Oklahoma City, OK

John W. Kusek, Ph.D.
Director, Urologic and Renal Clinical Trials Program
National Institute of Diabetes and
Digestive and Kidney Diseases
National Institutes of Health
Bethesda, MD

Edmund C. Lattime, Ph.D.
Associate Director
Cancer Institute of New Jersey
Professor of Surgery, Molecular Genetics,
and Microbiology
UMDNJ-Robert Wood Johnson Medical School
New Brunswick, NJ

James Lessard, Ph.D.
Professor
Division of Developmental Biology
Children's Hospital Medical Center
Cincinnati, OH

Robert M. Levin, Ph.D.
Director of Research
Office of Research Administration
Albany College of Medicine
Albany, NY

Monica Liebert, Ph.D.
Director, Office of Research
American Urological Association, Inc.
Baltimore, MD

Edward Macarak, Ph.D.
Professor
University of Pennsylvania
Philadelphia, PA

John D. McConnell, M.D.
Professor and Chairman
Department of Urology
University of Texas Southwestern Medical Center
Dallas, TX

Edward Messing, M.D.
Professor and Chairman
Department of Urology
University of Rochester Medical Center
Rochester, NY

Peggy Norton, M.D.
Associate Professor
Department of Obstetrics and Gynecology
University of Utah School of Medicine
Salt Lake City, UT

Leroy M. Nyberg, Jr., Ph.D., M.D.
Director, Urology Program
Division of Kidney, Urologic, and Hematologic Diseases
National Institute of Diabetes and
Digestive and Kidney Diseases
National Institutes of Health
Bethesda, MD

Vicki Ratner, M.D.
President, Interstitial Cystitis Association
Rockville, MD

Neil M. Resnick, M.D.
Professor and Chief
Division of Geriatric Medicine
Department of Medicine
University of Pittsburgh School of Medicine
Pittsburgh, PA

Brenda Russell, Ph.D.
Professor
Department of Physiology and Biophysics
University of Illinois at Chicago
Chicago, IL

Ricardo Saban, D.V.M., Ph.D.
Associate Professor
Department of Physiology
College of Medicine
University of Oklahoma
Oklahoma City, OK

Michael Sacks, Ph.D.
Assistant Professor
Department of Bioengineering
University of Pittsburgh
Pittsburgh, PA

Anthony J. Schaeffer, M.D.
Professor and Chair
Department of Urology
Northwestern University Medical School
Chicago, IL

Linda Dairiki Shortliffe, M.D.
Chair, Department of Urology
Stanford University School of Medicine
Stanford, CA

Michael B. Siroky, M.D.
Chief, Urology
Boston VA Medical Center
Boston, MA

Debra Slade, M.A.
President
National Bladder Foundation
Ridgefield, CT

Ann Stapleton, M.D.
Associate Professor of Medicine
University of Washington
Seattle, WA

William D. Steers, M.D.
Chair, Department of Urology
University of Virginia
Charlottesville, VA

Tung-Tien Sun, Ph.D.
Director
Department of Dermatology
New York University School of Medicine
New York, NY

Jeremy B. Tuttle, Ph.D.
Professor
Department of Neuroscience
University of Virginia
Charlottesville, VA

Dana Weaver-Osterholtz, M.D.
Clinical Associate Professor
University of Missouri
Columbia, MO

Anne Weber, M.D.
Project Officer
National Institute on Deafness and Other
Communication Disorders
National Institutes of Health
Bethesda, MD

Robert Weiss, M.D.
Professor and Chief
Section of Urology
Yale University School of Medicine
New Haven, CT

Ursula Wesselman, M.D.
Associate Professor
Department of Neurology/Neurosurgery
Johns Hopkins University School of Medicine
Baltimore, MD

INDEX

a

adhesin, 26, 124-125, 127, 130

aging *(see also elderly)*, 1, 3, 5-6, 9-10, 12-13, 19, 31, 33, 37-39, 42-43, 47, 54-57, 61, 64, 85-90, 93-94, 96, 98, 122, 136, 148, 151, 155, 157, 168, 197, 207

Alaskan Natives, 139

American Indian(s), 135-136, 139, 165

animal models, 8, 15, 22, 38, 47, 53, 55, 77, 89, 111, 126, 128, 130, 137, 148, 161, 166-168, 190, 192

anoxia, 55

antibiotic(s), 23-24, 27-28, 67, 72, 74, 78-79, 82, 104, 114, 120, 122-124, 130-131, 145

antibiotic resistance *(see also resistance)*, 24, 131

antimicrobial resistance *(see also resistance)*, 122, 125, 129, 131, 181

antiproliferative factor (APF), 106-110

apoptosis *(see also cell death)*

areflexia, 153

arrays *(see also microarrays)*, 22, 43, 56, 96, 118, 129, 162, 171-172, 192

Asian(s), Asian Americans, 68, 136, 165

attachment, 24, 124, 128

augmentation, 66-67, 71, 76, 188, 190

autoimmune, 58, 104-105

autologous cell transplantation, 44, 57

b

bacillus Calmette-Guerin (BCG), 107-108, 113, 167, 169

bacteremia, 120-122

bacterial invasion *(see also invasion)*, 24

bacteriuria, 66, 69, 118-123, 126, 128, 130, 139, 181

bedwetting *(see also enuresis)*, 65, 152, 164

benign prostatic hyperplasia (BPH), 10-11, 33-34, 43, 48, 85, 88, 93-96, 106, 137, 155, 181

bioengineering, 6, 15, 76, 88, 131, 177, 187, 190-191, 210-211

biofilm(s), 124-125, 131

bioinformatics, 7, 14-15, 22, 31, 56, 172, 177, 188, 191, 195-196

biomechanics, 9, 31, 41, 191, 207

biotechnology, 7, 15, 56, 99, 113, 129, 131, 177, 184, 197-198

birth *(see childbirth)*

bladder dysfunction, 5, 10, 34, 36, 41, 47, 53, 63, 65, 67-69, 76-78, 87, 89, 96-98, 106, 123, 134, 138-141, 183-185

blood sugar *(see also hyperglycemia)*, 123, 138-139, 144-145

blood supply, 9, 47-49, 51-52, 55, 72

blood vessels, 1, 7-9, 19, 32, 36, 41, 45, 47, 54, 57, 86, 95, 109, 134-135, 138-139, 149, 161, 198

blood in urine *(see also hematuria)*, 28, 174

bovine collagen, 44, 57

brain imaging, 9, 49, 58, 97

c

cancer, 1, 5-6, 9, 13-14, 21, 23-25, 27-29, 33, 43, 61, 85, 88, 91, 99, 104, 110, 130, 151, 161-175, 179-181, 187-191, 197, 203, 208-209

carcinogen(s), 21, 23, 28, 162, 165, 167, 169,

carcinogenesis, 165-167

catheter(s), 5, 11-12, 28-29, 82, 117, 119-122, 131, 162, 165, 199

catheterization, 5, 28-29, 66-67, 74, 119-122, 124, 153

Caucasian(s), 149, 161-163, 165, 171

cell-cell interactions, 21, 97, 128, 161

cell death, 24-25, 42, 52, 55, 126, 128, 161, 170

cell growth, 8, 22, 24-25, 191, 194

cell signaling, 8, 31-32, 34-36, 43, 124, 128, 135, 148, 155, 161, 165-166, 191, 193

ceramide pathway, 126

childbirth *(see also vaginal delivery, pelvic floor, pelvic floor trauma)*, 12-13, 31, 33, 39, 54, 148-150, 158, 179 children, 9-12, 17, 19, 23, 25, 34, 39, 44, 61, 63-76, 78, 80-83, 90-91, 93-94, 97, 100-101, 105, 115, 117-120, 135-136, 145, 150, 152, 155-156, 164, 189, 207, 209

colonization, 23, 71, 121, 125-126, 128, 130

congenital, 6, 10, 24, 63-65, 67-68, 70, 80, 93-94, 187, 189-190, 197

collagen, 8, 31-34, 42, 44, 57, 71, 95, 100, 148-149, 192

connective tissue, 1, 8, 15, 19, 31-39, 42, 87, 97, 139, 192, 198, 205

cystectomy, 28, 164, 189

cystopathy, 137, 144

cystoscopy, 14, 28, 75, 104, 107-108, 110, 112, 149, 162, 169-170

cytokines, 31-32, 37, 126-128, 130, 165, 169, 193

cytotoxic necrotizing factor (CNF), 124, 128-129

diabetes, 1, 3, 5-7, 9, 12-13, 17, 19, 27, 31, 33, 39, 41, 43, 48, 52-53, 55, 61, 64, 88, 106, 117-120, 123, 133-145, 148, 152-153, 157, 179-180, 183, 197-198, 201, 203, 207-209

diabetic bladder, 1, 13, 52, 55, 134, 137, 141, 153, 180

differentiation, 8, 14, 21-22, 24-25, 36-37, 112, 141, 161, 191-193

dysfunctional voiding (see also voiding dysfunction), 10, 64-65, 68-69, 79, 89, 152

ectopic ureters, 65, 75, 79

Escherichia coli, E. coli, 23-25, 121, 123-130

effector, 9, 41, 169

elastin, 31-34, 42

elderly *(see also aging)*, 11-12, 17, 54, 61, 87-90, 96, 117, 119-120, 122, 136, 145, 149, 151-153, 156, 159, 161-163, 165, 170-171, 175

endoderm, 24, 35

end-stage bladder failure, 42-43, 97

enuresis *(see also bedwetting)*, 63, 65, 68-70, 79, 149, 152

enzymes, 32, 37

eosinophils, 27

epidemiology, 1, 5-8, 13, 21-27, 32, 34-38, 43-44, 51, 77, 88-89, 95, 107, 109-110, 112, 127-128, 130, 134, 148, 162, 166-168, 172, 174, 191-193, 195, 198, 205

epigenetics, 86

epispadias, 70-71, 152

epithelium (urothelium), 1, 5-8, 13, 19, 32, 34-38, 43-44, 51, 77, 95, 107, 109-110, 112, 127-128, 130, 134, 148, 166-168, 172, 174, 191-193, 195, 198, 205

estrogen, 33, 54, 77, 89, 105, 123, 149-150

exfoliation, 24, 126-127

exstrophy, 1, 5, 10, 61, 64-65, 70-72, 76, 80, 152

female(s) *(see also women)*, 13, 23, 32, 35-36, 48, 50, 54, 70-71, 74, 78, 87, 89-90, 98, 105, 117-118, 134, 149

fiber, 31, 33-34, 195

field effect, 14, 23, 161, 165

fibrosis, 34, 71, 73, 164

fimbria, fimbriae *(see also pili)*, 24, 124-126, 128

FimH, 26, 124-125, 127, 130

Franklin, Benjamin, 1, 5, 199

frequency *(see also urinary frequency)*, 10-11, 43, 48, 50, 64, 69, 93, 103-107, 112-115, 123, 144-145, 152-153, 198

gene expression, 22, 34-38, 110, 125, 166, 168, 190, 192, 194-196

gene therapy, 8, 15, 44, 47-49, 53, 57, 134, 136, 141, 166, 177, 181, 190-191, 194, 196

genomics, 7-8, 15, 34-38, 48-49, 52, 56, 96, 125, 127, 129, 148, 166, 171, 175, 177, 187-188, 190-192, 194, 196-198

glomerulations, 104, 107, 114

glucose, 88, 124, 138-140, 144-145

glycocalyx, 22

glycosoaminoglycans (GAG), 22, 25

glycososphingolipids (GSL), 128

glycosuria, 139

glycosylation, 138

growth factor(s), 21, 25-26, 31-32, 35-36, 42, 47, 53, 77, 87-89, 95, 98, 104-105, 107-110, 138, 140, 148-149, 161, 165, 168-169, 191, 193, 194-195

growth-factor-binding protein, 109

growth-modulating factors, 22

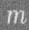

muscle, 1, 8-9, 19, 26, 28, 31-38, 41-45, 50-53, 55, 57-59, 68-69, 71, 73, 76-77, 86-91, 95, 97, 100-101, 115, 122-123, 134, 137, 148, 151-155, 158-159, 164, 170, 174, 181, 189, 191-195, 205

muscle dysfunction, 43

muscle failure, 41-43

myelodysplasia (see also spina bifida), 10, 64-65, 78

myelomeningocele, 76, 93-94, 152

n

nephropathy, 66, 74, 139-140, 143

nerve(s), 1, 7-9, 9, 21, 26, 32, 36, 42-43, 45, 47-49, 51-58, 63, 65-66, 74, 80, 86, 88, 105, 108, 111, 113, 115, 122, 133-134, 135, 137-139, 140, 144-145, 148, 153-154, 158, 164, 194, 198, 205

neurogenic, neurogenic bladder, 1, 7, 10, 12, 35-36, 47, 53, 58-59, 63, 65, 69, 85, 104-105, 107, 111, 162, 181

neuromodulation, 9, 45, 89

neuropathic, neuropathic bladder, 33, 97, 141, 144, 152

neuropathy, 12, 55, 133, 137-141, 144-145, 153

neurostimulation, 115

neurotransmitters, 26, 53, 111

neurotrophic, 47, 49, 51-52, 55, 111, 141

nitric oxide, 23, 26, 56, 76, 107, 111, 140

nighttime voiding (see also nocturia), 10, 59, 69, 88, 93, 152

nocturia (see also nighttime voiding), 10, 59, 69, 88, 90, 93, 152, 164

o

obesity, 135-136, 139, 149, 151, 155

obstruction, 1, 5, 7, 9-11, 31, 33-37, 43, 49, 53, 56, 61, 63-67, 69, 72, 75, 79, 85-86, 88, 93-99, 121, 123, 149, 151, 167, 179-181, 188, 198, 204

oncogenes, 22, 24, 168, 191

p

Parkinson's disease, 5, 11, 13, 35-36, 41, 48, 64, 103, 105, 148, 152-153

Parkinsonism, 43

pathogenicity islands, 125, 128-129

pelvic floor, 1, 15, 32-33, 37-38, 43, 50, 59, 69, 71, 77, 87, 90, 109, 135, 150, 154-156, 158-159, 187-190, 192-198

pelvic organ prolapse, 31, 33, 38-39, 89, 135-136, 156-157

permeability, 21, 25-27, 104-105, 108

P fimbriae, 124, 126, 128

pharmacology, 1, 9, 15, 41, 89, 155, 187, 198, 201, 206, 208

pili, 23-25, 124-128, 130

polymerase chain reaction (PCR), 175, 190

posterior urethral valves (PUV), 1, 10, 61, 63-65, 67-68, 76, 79, 82, 93-95, 100

post-prostatectomy incontinence, 1, 34, 88, 90-91

pregnancy, 12-13, 39, 80-81, 100, 118, 120-122

probiotics, 130

prostate, 22, 24, 28, 33-34, 43, 73, 75, 85-86, 88, 90-91, 93-94, 96, 99, 106, 119, 122-123, 134, 140, 149, 151, 157, 166, 171, 173, 190

prostate cancer, 33, 43, 85, 88, 151, 171, 173, 190

prostatectomy, 88, 90, 151, 153, 155

prostatitis, 88, 103, 105-106, 119, 135

proteomics, 7-8, 15, 22, 34-38, 48-49, 52, 56, 110, 127, 129, 148, 162, 166-167, 171, 175, 177, 188, 191-192

prune belly syndrome, 10, 64-65, 72-74, 79

pyelonephritis (see also kidney infection), 12, 23, 67, 74, 121-123

P53, 167, 175

q

quorum sensing, 125

r

receptors, 15, 23-26, 35-37, 53, 77, 89, 111-112, 124, 126-128, 130, 177, 193

reflux (see also vesicoureteral reflux), 1, 9-10, 23-25, 27, 44, 59, 61, 63-67, 69, 71-74, 76, 78, 81-83, 94, 97, 100, 121, 187-188

regeneration, 8-9, 34-36, 42, 47, 49, 51, 55, 135, 188, 191, 193, 195-196, 198

renal scarring (see also hypertension), 66-67, 83

reperfusion, 51-52, 55, 96

repositories, 22, 99, 143

resistance (see also antibiotic and antimicrobial), 24, 97, 122, 125, 128-129, 131, 135, 137, 181

reservoirs, 125-127, 129, 164, 188

retention (see also urinary retention), 5, 9, 12, 41-43, 58, 69, 74, 93, 133, 137-138, 151, 153, 164

s

serotonin, 51, 53

smoking, 55, 145, 164-165, 167, 169, 171, 175

specimen banks, 99, 131, 142, 155, 157, 171-172, 184-185, 197

sphincter, 19, 33, 37, 41-44, 48, 50, 57, 68-69, 71-72, 74-75, 77, 85-88, 91, 138-139, 151-152, 154, 192

spina bifida *(see also myelodysplasia)*, 5, 10, 63-66, 78, 93-94, 120, 152

spinal cord injury, 5, 13, 39, 43, 47-49, 53, 93-94, 121, 148, 152-153

stem cells, 37, 42, 141, 177, 187-191, 193-194, 196-198

stress incontinence, 35-36, 44, 57, 138-139, 148-150, 154, 157, 164

stress response, 125

stroke, 6, 19, 41, 43, 50-51, 57, 144, 152

t

Tamm-Horsfall, 25

tissue banks, 16, 22, 27, 78, 90, 98-99, 113, 143, 162, 171-172

tissue engineering, 8, 15, 44, 49, 53, 57, 77, 89, 177, 187-189, 191, 193-194, 196-198

tissue recombination, 24, 35

toxins, 21-23, 25, 28, 52, 124, 161, 175

transduction, 41, 107

transgenic(s), 22, 26-27, 47, 49, 53, 166, 168

transplant *(see also kidney transplant)*, 5, 26, 47, 53, 100-101, 124

trigone, 24, 75

tumor-host interaction, 169

type 1-fimbriated (piliated), 23-25, 124, 127-128

u

ureterocele, 74-75, 79

ureterostomy, 101

urethra, 15, 19, 24, 33-34, 42, 44-45, 48, 57, 64, 67, 70-75, 82, 85-87, 89, 91, 95, 100-101, 134, 137, 141, 148-149, 151, 154, 159, 164, 184-185, 187-191, 193-196

urge incontinence, 10, 44, 47, 53, 138, 149, 151-154

urgency, 10-11, 43, 50, 64, 68, 93, 103, 105, 107, 112-115, 144-145, 151-153, 198

urinary diversion, 28, 72, 74, 97, 163-164, 175

urinary

urinary frequency *(see also frequency)*, 93, 105, 114, 144-145

urinary incontinence *(see also incontinence)*, 1, 5, 9, 12-13, 33, 38-39, 44, 48-49, 54, 57, 61, 65, 67-69, 78-79, 85-90, 93-94, 135, 138-141, 147-148, 150-157, 159, 187-189

urinary retention *(see also retention)*, 5, 9, 12, 58, 69, 93, 137-138, 151, 153, 164

urinary tract infection (UTI) *(see also infection)*, 1, 11-12, 23-24, 58, 65-66, 69-70, 75-76, 82, 86, 93, 100, 103-104, 119, 125, 127, 134, 144-145, 152, 164, 181

urinary urgency *(see also urgency)*, 11, 68, 103, 107, 113, 115, 198

uropathogens, uropathogenic, 22, 25, 120-121, 124-130

uroplakin(s), 24-26, 77, 89, 168

urothelium *(see also epithelium)*, 1, 13, 21-27, 35-36, 88-89, 95, 162, 165, 167-168

v

vaccine(s), 12, 24, 127, 130, 168

vaginal delivery *(see also childbirth)*, 33, 42-43, 150, 154-155, 158

valves *(see also vesicoureteral valves)*, 1, 10, 61, 63-65, 67-68, 76, 79, 82, 93-95, 100-101

vesicoureteral reflux *(see also reflux)*, 1, 9-10, 23-25, 27, 44, 61, 63-67, 69, 71, 73, 76, 78, 81-82, 94, 121, 188

virulence factors, 124-126, 128

voiding dysfunction *(see also dysfunctional voiding)*, 11, 41-43, 51, 54, 68-69, 93-94, 97, 152-153, 181

vulvodynia, 105, 109, 114

w

women (see also female), 5-6, 10-13, 23, 35, 38-39, 51, 54-55, 61, 85-89, 91, 96, 103-106, 113, 117-120, 122-125, 130-131, 133-136, 138-141, 147, 149-151, 154-155, 158-159, 161-165, 171, 175, 184, 207

workforce, 16, 27, 90, 98, 113, 131, 142, 155, 184, 196

x

xenograft, 167

www.ingramcontent.com/pod-product-compliance
Lightning Source LLC
Chambersburg PA
CBHW081440170526
45166CB00008B/2259